Empathy in the Helping Relationship

Ruth C. MacKay, RN, PhD was Professor at the School of Nursing at Dalhousie University in Halifax, Canada for the past 12 years. She has a B.A. in Arts and Nursing from McMaster University, an M.N. and M.A. in sociology from Emory University, and a Ph.D. in medical behavioral sciences from the University of Kentucky. She has taught nursing and research methods at Dalhousie, Mc-Master, and Queens Universities in Canada, and previous to that at the University of Kentucky and Emory. During her tenure at Dalhousie she developed the Nursing Research Department at the Victoria General Hospital in Halifax. She has published and given papers both nationally and internationally. Currently she is Principal Lecturer at the School of Nursing of the Western Australian College of Advanced Education, teaching in the graduate and undergraduate programs, and co-ordinator, Nursing Research, at Sir Charles Gairdner Hospital in Perth, Australia.

Jean R. Hughes, RN, MS is an Associate Professor at Dalhousie University where she teaches interaction theory and its application in both the undergraduate and graduate nursing programs. She obtained a Master's degree in Community Mental Health and Psychiatric Nursing from Boston University. Her clinical practice focuses on the interaction process of single mothers, known to have a high potential for abuse, and their pre-school children. Her involvement in the Professional Nursing Association at the provincial and national levels is very active. She has written and collaborated on a number of articles and chapters in a book and has presented scholarly papers at local, regional, national, and international meetings.

E. Joyce Carver, RN, BN, MEd is an Assistant Professor at Dalhousie University, School of Nursing in Halifax. She obtained a Master's degree in educational media and technology from Boston University. Her special areas of interest include the use of video technology to teach helping relationship skills and the development of learning laboratories. Her practice area is in community health nursing. She has taught at all levels in the undergraduate generic nursing baccalaureate program and has coordinated the post-RN baccalaureate program. She has written and collaborated on several articles and presented research and scholarly papers at local, regional and national conferences. She is currently on study leave to pursue a doctoral degree in educational administration at the University of British Columbia.

Empathy in the Helping Relationship

Ruth C. MacKay, RN., Ph.D.
Jean R. Hughes, R.N., M.S.
E. Joyce Carver, R.N., B.N., M.Ed.

Editors

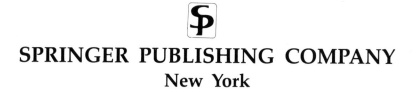

SPRINGER PUBLISHING COMPANY
New York

Copyright © 1990 by Springer Publishing Company, Inc.

Springer Publishing Company, Inc.
536 Broadway
New York, NY 10012

90 91 93 94 95 / 5 4 3 2 1

Library of Congress Cataloging-in-Publication Data

Empathy in the helping relationship / Ruth C. MacKay, Jean R.
    Hughes, E. Joyce Carver, editors.
        p.   cm.
    Includes bibliographies and index.
    ISBN 0-8261-6140-5
    1. Nursing—Psychological aspects.   2. Nurse and patient.
3. Empathy.   I. MacKay, Ruth C.   II. Hughes, Jean R.   III. Carver,
E. Joyce.
        [DNLM: 1. Empathy.   2. Helping Behavior.   BF 575.E55 E555]
RT86.E56   1989
610.73'06'99—dc20
DNLM/DLC
for Library of Congress   89–11408
                                                                              CIP

Printed in the United States of America

To the nurses on Seven North at the Victoria General Hospital in Halifax who courageously participated in the research reported here, and volunteered to have their communication with patients examined so that other health professionals might benefit.

Contents

Foreword

Empathy is the focus of this important publication. The authors view empathy as a distinguishing characteristic at the heart of helping relationships. For the past three decades, there has been considerable scientific interest and inquiry into the nature of this intriguing phenomenon. The editors of this textbook, three Canadian nurse-scholars, present their own significant work and that of invited contributors toward clarification of the nature of empathy. Publications of many other scholars and researchers have also been reviewed and summarized for inclusion in this text. All of these efforts are directed toward achieving greater understanding and scientific validity of theory related to empathy.

Helping relationships are fundamental in the provision of health services, particularly professional nursing practice. The day is already past when such relationships were guided solely by good intentions. Today, professionals are expected to know and to apply the most well-defined and rigorously researched scientific concepts germane to the work for which their service is being provided. This textbook provides a wide array of useful, current information on the concept of empathy and on its significance in helping relationships.

Clients seek help from professionals out of necessity, in order to understand and to resolve problems related to their health status. At such times, the expectations of clients are that the professionals will be competent and will have the knowledge required to explain and to solve the client's presenting difficulties. Furthermore, and of equal if not greater importance, clients expect that professionals will be sensitive to their personal reactions to these changes or dilemmas in their lives. Professionals are expected to recognize and respond humanely to the changing human condition of clients during the helping relationship. Thus, competence, knowledge, and sensitivity are three critical features in effective helping relationships. This edited volume describes and defines empathy from these three major standpoints.

Empathy is an intriguing and yet elusive phenomenon. The basic question addressed in this work is: What is empathy? Is it an innate ability or a learned skill? Is empathy an attitude or a value? Is it largely a cognitive process of sensing, perceiving, observing, thinking and knowing, or is it largely a behavioral process or way of acting and doing? Is empathy an emotional phenomenon in which one person experiences the feelings another person is having, or is it a cognitive understanding of the situation of another person? Is empathy akin to intuition or is it an insight; that is, is it a process of sensing or is it a product of inferring? Is it merely a guess if the product of empathizing is not validated by the person who is the subject of the empathy? Is empathy as individual ability that has utility only in interpersonal situations? Must the other person be present or can there be physical distance between the empathizer and the subject or subjects? Does empathy occur in different degrees—such as lower or higher levels—and, if so, what reliable measures determine these differences? Can empathy be "given" by one person to another? In other words, is empathy a phenomenon that can and should be narrowly defined, or is there merit and scientific evidence for a broad, all-encompassing definition of empathy as a multi-faceted concept? There are many questions about the nature of empathy. The authors of various chapters in this book explore the foregoing issues and present their own position based upon contemporary knowledge about empathy.

This work is a significant contribution to an enlarging literature. It presents an historical review, a comprehensive overview of current viewpoints on empathy, cogent analysis, and it also suggests practical applications of the current knowledge. The authors provide for their readers a broad scope of contemporary definitions of the nature of empathy. This text directs the attention of students, their teachers, practicing professionals, and researchers to what is known about empathy at this point in time, and toward the unresolved issues which merit further study. This work therefore is intended simultaneously to inform the readers and to involve them in further debate or investigation of empathy. It is a timely work on an important subject.

HILDEGARD E. PEPLAU, R.N., F.A.A.N
Professor Emerita
Rutgers, The State University of New Jersey

Acknowledgments

We wish to thank the many individuals who have contributed to the Empathy Study Program reported in this book, and to our exploration of empathy as an important factor in helping relationships. The nurses on the Seven North Nursing Unit at the Victoria General Hospital in Halifax, Nova Scotia started us on the way with their interest in improving the care of patients on their unit. Ruth E. Dennison, at that time Associate Director of Nursing at the Victoria General Hospital, facilitated the beginning study of nurse–patient communication on Seven North. Subsequently Marlene A. Grantham, Director of Nursing, has offered continued encouragement, and has developed a climate which is supportive of health care research. Christine Heggelin and Nora Gene Goodwin, Head Nurses on Seven North during the study period, gave unselfishly of their thought, energy, and time in contributing clinical information and in smoothing the research process. Critical to the research, we thank the patients on Seven North who agreed to participate.

Our contributing authors have provided discussions of empathy from specialized perspectives, and we thank them for their scholarly achievements. Additionally, we are grateful to a number of colleagues who reviewed drafts of various chapters, making helpful suggestions: Margaret Bayer, Barbara Keddy, Jacquelyn Peitchinis, Judith Ritchie, Denise Sommerfeld, Phyllis Stern, Miriam Stewart, Patricia Sullivan, and Deborah Tamlyn. In particular, we wish to thank Elaine La Monica who reviewed the manuscript. Her cogent observations prompted several adjustments. We are grateful to her for her effort and skill.

The typing of the manuscript has rested heavily on Wanda Hunter and Joan Hutchinson, and on Pat Hoag who facilitated the secretarial services from the School of Nursing. We appreciate their skill and care in the completion of this book.

We acknowledge the Dalhousie University School of Nursing Research and Development Fund and the Dalhousie University Faculty of Graduate Studies for financial assistance in some phases of the Empathy Study Program. Also, we are grateful to George M. Gazda and Allyn and Bacon, Publishers, for permission to copy the Empathy Scale published in 1975 in *Human Relations Development* by George M. Gazda, Richard P. Walters, and William C. Childers.

Ruth C. MacKay
Jean R. Hughes
E. Joyce Carver

Contributors

Bryn D. Davis, S.R.N., R.M.N., R.N.T., S.Sc., Ph.D. is Principal Lecturer in Nursing Studies, Department of Community Studies, Brighton Polytechnic, Brighton, England.

Timothy D. Evans, Ph.D., Educational Program Specialist, College of Education, at the University of Georgia

George M. Gazda, Ed.D., is Research Professor of Education and Associate Dean for Research at the University of Georgia, and Clinical Professor of Psychiatry at the Medical College of Georgia.

John A. Johnson, M.A., Ph.D., is Assistant Professor, Department of Psychology, Pennsylvania State University, DuBois Campus.

Jacquelyn Peitchinis, R.N., B.Sc.N., M.Phil., M.Sc., Ph.D., C. Psych., is Director of Nursing Research, Calgary District Hospital Group in Calgary Canada and Adjunct Assistant Professor in Community Health Sciences and Psychiatry at the Faculty of Medicine, the University of Calgary.

Part I

Empathy as a Concept

The study of empathy has been going on for a number of decades and from several perspectives. Although there is some general consensus on the nature of empathy, there are marked differences in how it is conceptualized. Changing patterns of health care increasingly require helping relationship skills from professionals. Moreover, the introduction of high levels of technology into health care needs to be balanced with humanistic, caring interactions. Chapter 1 explores the various conceptualizations of empathy revealed in the published literature, and Chapter 2 discusses the significance of empathy for professional practice. In Chapter 3, Peitchinis reviews the origins of the study of empathy: what prompted this interest, how it developed, and how this affected the study of empathy today.

1

What Is Empathy?

Ruth C. MacKay

Effective interpersonal communication skills are central to the provision of quality client care in health and social services (Gazda, Walters, & Childers, 1975; La Monica, Wolf, Madea, & Oberst, 1987; Peitchinis, 1976; Peplau, 1952). Helping professionals need to hear what the client says, and need to validate the inferred meaning of this with the client (Joel & Collins, 1978, p. 89; Orlando, 1961; Wolf, Woolliscroft, Calhoun, & Boxer, 1987). This process leads to the identification of the client's perception of need and paves the way for mutual planning of interventions, relevant to resolution of the client's problem. A basic component of effective communication is the helping professional's ability to make empathic responses to the client, responses which reveal an understanding of the client's statements and an attitude of caring, critical to a helping relationship.

Behavioral scientists, developmental psychologists, counseling psychologists, psychotherapists, and health care practitioners have identified different ways of looking at empathy as a factor of importance in interpersonal relations and the helping relationship. This chapter discusses various ways in which empathy is conceptualized and defined. Later chapters address other questions related to empathy in the helping relationship: theoretical issues, measurement problems, the professional's ability to be empathic, and the effects of the professional's use of empathy on client outcomes.

EMPATHY CONCEPTUALIZED

Practitioners and scientists conceptualize empathy fundamentally in three ways. One is a behavioral approach. The observed behavior of the professional in interaction with a client can be viewed as the revealing of ability to use empathy with higher or lower degrees of proficiency. Another approach is a personality perspective of empathy. The values, attitudes, or personality orientations of helping professionals influence their natural tendency to be or not to be empathic. A third fundamental conceptualization is found in the work of those who view empathy as experiencing the emotions of others. The helping professional responds to viewing the client's situation with an emotional reaction somewhat similar to the emotion revealed by the client. The affective quality of the interaction appears to be contagious. Some writers draw on more than one kind of conceptualization. Moreover, proponents of any one of these perspectives may not necessarily acknowledge the value of others' conceptualizations in explaining the influence of empathy in therapeutic communication.

Empathy as a Behavior

In considering empathy as a behavior there is the assumption that the helping professional's observed behavior is indicative of empathy. In addition, observed behavior is perceived differently depending on the role of the observer. First of all, empathic behavior can be viewed by an independent observer. But alternatively, the professional's empathic behavior can be perceived by others concerned in the process of communication: the client, the professional's peers, and the professional looking at self. Thus the concept of empathy changes accordingly. Let us examine each of these variations.

Observed empathy

Rogers (1975), Carkhuff (1969), Gazda (1982), and Gazda and his colleagues (1975), to mention a few, have discussed empathy as a basic and critical component of the helping relationship. Gazda et al. state that "empathy is the attempt by a helper to 'tune in' to the feelings of a helpee" (1975, p. 55). The helper's behavior is observed by an independent observer in this "tuning in" process. Aspy (1975) sees empathy "as the ability to understand and to communicate to another your understanding of both his feeling and the reasons for his feeling" (p. 11). Behavior demonstrating empathy in the communication process is observed by an observer external to the communication.

Orlando (1972) describes a process of verification in a therapeutic encounter which could be likened to observed empathy. She suggests verification of the meaning of observations with the patient is one of three crucial elements in a process discipline. She believes nurses must have their perceptions validated or corrected in order for "understanding of one's own and another's immediate experience" (p. 32), which is basic to empathic behavior.

Peplau (1952) speaks indirectly about empathy in her comments about nursing care. "Understanding of the meaning of the experience to the patient is required in order for nursing to function as an educative, therapeutic, maturing force" (p. 41).

Perceived empathy

A number of behavioral scientists and helping professionals seek to identify empathy as a component of communication which can be described by the persons involved. One of the most well-known approaches is put forth by Barrett-Lennard (1962) who discusses the "received empathy, or empathy based on the experience of the person empathized with" (1981, p. 95) which is generally called *client-perceived empathy*. Kunst-Wilson, Carpenter, Poser, Venohr, and Kushner (1981) have conceptualized empathy as the ability to judge the feelings of others (p. 286) which can be inferred by an independent observer or by the helping professional involved. Judgements by peers also have been used as an adjunct or alternative to observations by an independent observer (D'Augelli, 1973; Kalisch, 1971; La Monica, 1981). These conceptual variations of perceived empathy will be discussed further when the operationalization of empathy is addressed in the chapter on measurement (Chapter 7).

Empathy as a Personality Dimension

Many psychologists and investigators in the area of human relations view empathy as a dimension of the individual's personality. (See, for example, Dagenais & Meleis, 1982; Davis, 1983; Feshbach, 1975; Hogan, 1969, 1975; Iannotti, 1975; Kerr, 1960.) Hogan offers a rather general perspective. He discusses an empathic disposition, stating it is the "capacity to adopt a broad moral perspective, that is, to take 'the moral point of view' " (1969, p. 307). Conceptualizing empathy in terms of the roles individuals take in relation to each other while in interaction, he writes that "empathy refers to the process of representing to oneself the expectations that others hold with regard to one's behavior." (1975, p. 15). This statement is perhaps too broad for empirical use and Hogan bypasses further concern at the conceptual level and operationalizes empathy in a scale which has been used extensively by others. Forsyth (1979), who used Hogan's scale in the examination of the empathy of nurses, gives this interpretation: "Empathic individuals are those who possess keen insight, imaginative perceptiveness and social acuity about other persons" (p. 55).

Steibe, Boulet, and Lee (1979) conceptualize empathy as having two components. One is *trait empathy* which is viewed as a natural empathic disposition and a relatively stable personality dimension. The other is *state empathy*, an ability which can be trained and is revealed as an interpersonal skill (p. 42). The state empathy appears to be similar to the behavioral conceptualization of empathy. The trait empathy, on the other hand, falls squarely in the realm of personality.

Dagenais and Meleis (1982) identify a personality dimension they entitle *empathy*, which has as subdimensions adaptability, sociability, consideration, and sensitivity (p. 415). In general, however, empathy as a personality dimension has suffered from problems of conceptualization and a lack of consensus. Iannotti (1975) has remarked upon this lack of agreement among writers and suggests that "empathy in its broadest sense refers to the responsiveness of an individual to the feelings of another person" (p. 22).

Empathy as Experienced Emotion

Several investigators view empathy as the ability to experience the emotions of others. Stotland, Mathews, Sherman, Hansson, and Richardson (1978) write that empathy can be described as an emotional reaction to the perceived experiences of another (p. 7). They assert that when an individual experiences an emotion which is somewhat similar to another's (recognizing that it is impossible for it to be identical to another's experience) the emotion can be termed empathy (p. 12). They state that empathy is influenced by all the factors in a social situation, such as the perceived similarity of the participants, their status, and their previous interaction history, as well as the personal orientation of the empathizer (p. 27).

Batson, and others who have written with him, approach empathy as an emotion which can affect motivation to help another (Batson, Coke, & Pych, 1983; Batson, O'Quin, Vanderplas, & Isen, 1983; Coke, Batson, & McDavis, 1978; Toi & Batson, 1982). Their two-stage model of empathic mediation of helping involves the individual in (a) taking the perspective of a person in need which produces an empathic emotional response, with (b) the emotion in turn acting to motivate a helping stance to reduce the need in the other (Coke et al., 1978, p. 753). Empathy, then, takes on the properties of a feeling. Archer, Diaz-Loving, Gollwitzer, Davis, & Foushee (1981) propose that dispositional and situational factors enter this two-stage process as well. Batson and his colleagues make a distinction between personal distress which leads to egoistic motivation, and empathy which leads to altruistic motivation (Batson, O'Quin, Vanderplas, & Isen, 1983).

Feshbach (1975) puts forward a three-component model of empathy. Two of these components are cognitive: "the ability to discriminate the perspective and role of another person," and cognitive competence. The third component is emotional capacity and responsiveness (p. 26). Feshbach states that an emotional response to a situation requires all three components. Moreover, empathy is seen to vary with the experiences of the perceiving individual and with progress in the individual's psychosocial development as well.

One other approach to conceptualizing empathy as experienced emotion is given by Mehrabian and Epstein (1972). They have visualized empathy as an emotion (p. 526) derived from experiencing the imagined emotions of another as perceived from observed behavior (p. 525). The operationalization of their concept of empathy into a measure of empathic tendency has been used frequently by a number of investigators. As an example, Barnett, Howard, King, and Dino (1981) used the measure to discriminate ability to be empathically aroused. They showed a videotaped presentation on handicapped children, suited for viewing by adolescents, to high school students. Following the presentation the experimental situation allowed opportunity for participant viewers of the tape to make activity booklets for the use of handicapped institutionalized children. Students viewing the presentation who had scored above the median in empathic tendency made more activity booklets for handicapped children than did those who had scored lower in empathic tendency. The conclusion reached was that highly empathic adolescents demonstrated more helpful behavior than those who showed lower empathic tendency.

The process of indirect experiences producing an emotion resulting from the observation of another suggests there may be a relationship between empathy and sympathy. The distinction has not always been made apparent in the various conceptualizations.

Empathy and Sympathy

Several authors have discussed empathy as it is similar to, yet different from, sympathy. Szalita (1976) makes a distinction, introducing McKellar's definition of empathy. Placing oneself in the shoes of another permits sympathetic understanding of the other's mental life. However, empathy in this case is understanding, rather than "siding with" (p. 145). Rogers (1975) is careful to keep empathy in the realm of perceiving the other "as if" he were the other, but remembering to retain this "as if" condition (p. 3).

Gazda and associates (1975) express the differentiation quite clearly.

> Empathy and sympathy are different. Sympathy means that the helper experiences the same emotions as the helpee. . . . Fortunately, it is not necessary to experience the helpee's feelings to be helpful. You can help if you can understand how the other person feels, and that is what is meant by empathy. (p. 56)

Empirical evidence of a distinction between empathy and sympathy is offered by Gruen and Mendelsohn (1986) who found empathy to be a stable personality factor, whereas sympathy depended on an interaction between the personality of the observer and the plight of the individual in the observed situation.

Travelbee (1966), on the other hand, views sympathy as genuine concern for the client coupled with a desire to help the client in alleviating distress (p. 146). Her discussion of sympathy as "warmth, kindness, a transient type of compassion, a *caring* quality experienced on a feeling level and communicated to another" (p. 147) shows it to be somewhat similar to empathy as conceptualized by others.

Thus the distinction between empathy and sympathy maintained by some writers is not necessarily accepted by others, and there is ambiguity in the use of terms.

EMPATHY DEFINED

It should not be surprising to find as many definitions of empathy as there are conceptualizations. Some examples show the variations in types to be found.

Proponents of the behavioral model define empathy as an ability. Valle's (1981) definition is typical. "Empathy is the ability to respond to the feelings and reasons for the feelings the patient is experiencing in a manner that communicates an understanding of the patient" (p. 784). La Monica (1981) notes the confusion revealed in the literature concerning an adequate operational definition of empathy, and provides the following: "Empathy signifies a central focus and feeling *with* and *in* the client's world by the helper, communication of this understanding to the client, and the client's perception of the helper's understanding" (p. 398).

Authors who view empathy from the perspective of one who is involved in the communication process adopt a different kind of definition. Barrett-Lennard's (1962) definition has been cited frequently: "Degree of empathic understanding is conceived as the extent to which one person is conscious of the immediate awareness of another" (p. 3).

Different again, followers of the model of empathy as a personality dimension define empathy in terms of its affect. Iannotti (1975) writes "Empathy in its broadest sense refers to the responsiveness of an individual to the feelings of another person" (p. 22). When empathy is seen as experienced emotion, the definition reflects this perspective. Namie (1982/1983), as example, states that "Empathy is the ability to experience the emotions of others as if they are one's own."

SUMMARY

As the examination of empathy proceeds, both in the published literature, and in the discussions put forward in this book, definitions of empathy will differ, according to the conceptualizations involved in the arguments presented. Is one conceptualization of empathy superior to another? The chapters to follow will argue this point, offering evidence for support as this is available.

This chapter has discussed the meaning of empathy from three conceptual perspectives: as a behavior, as a personality dimension, and as the experienced emotion of another. Typical definitions of empathy reflective of these perspectives were given, and some distinctions between empathy and sympathy were reviewed.

REFERENCES

Archer, R. L., Diaz-Loving, R., Gollwitzer, P. M., Davis M. H., & Foushee, H. C. (1981). The role of dispositional empathy and social evaluation in the empathic mediation of helping. *Journal of Personality and Social Psychology, 40,* 786–796.

Aspy, D. N. (1975). Empathy: Let's get the hell on with it. *The Counseling Pychologist, 5*(2), 10–14.

Barnett, M. A., Howard, J. A., King, L. M., & Dino, G. A. (1981). Helping behavior and the transfer of empathy. *The Journal of Social Psychology, 115,* 125–132.

Barrett-Lennard, G. T. (1962). Dimensions of therapist response as causal factors in therapeutic change. *Psychological Monographs, 76* (43, Whole No. 562).

Barrett-Lennard, G. T. (1981). The empathy cycle: Refinement of a nuclear concept. *Journal of Counseling Psychology, 28,* 91–100.

Batson, C. D., Coke, J. S., & Pych, V. (1983). Limits on the two-stage model of empathic mediation of helping: A reply to Archer, Diaz-Loving, Gollwitzer, & Foushee. *Journal of Personality and Social Psychology, 45,* 895–898.

Batson, C. D., O'Quin, K., Fultz, J., Vanderplas, M., & Isen, A. M. (1983). Influence of self-reported distress and empathy on egoistic versus altruistic motivation to help. *Journal of Personality and Social Psychology, 45,* 706–718.

Carkhuff, R. R. (1969). *Helping and human relations: A primer for lay and professional helpers.* Vols. 1 & 2. New York: Holt, Rinehart, & Winston.

Coke, J. S., Batson, C. D., & McDavis, K. (1978). Empathic mediation of helping: A two-stage model. *Journal of Personality and Social Psychology, 36,* 752–766.

Dagenais, F., & Meleis, A. I. (1982). Professionalism, work ethic, and empathy in nursing: The Nurse Self-Description Form. *Western Journal of Nursing Research, 4,* 407–422.

D'Augelli, A. R. (1973). The assessment of interpersonal skills: A comparison of observer, peer, and self-ratings. *Journal of Community Psychology, 1,* 177–179.

Davis, M. H. (1983). The effects of dispositional empathy on emotional reactions and helping: A multidimensional approach. *Journal of Personality, 51,* 167–184.

Elizur, A., & Rosenheim, E. (1982). Empathy and attitudes among medical students: The effects of group experience. *Journal of Medical Education, 57,* 675–683.

Feshbach, N. D. (1975). Empathy in children: Some theoretical and empirical considerations. *The Counseling Psychologist, 5*(2), 25–30.

Forsyth, G. L. (1979). Exploration of empathy in nurse–client interaction. *Advances in Nursing Science, 1*(2), 53–61.

Gazda, G. M., Childers, W. C., & Walters, R. P. (1982). *Interpersonal communication.* Rockville, MD: Aspen.

Gazda, G. M., Walters, R. P., & Childers, W. C. (1975). *Human relations development: A manual for health sciences.* Boston: Allyn & Bacon.

Gruen, R. J., & Mendelsohn, G. (1986). Emotional responses to affective displays in others: The distinction between empathy and sympathy. *Journal of Personality and Social Psychology, 51,* 609–614.

Hogan, R. (1969). Development of an empathy scale. *Journal of Consulting and Clinical Psychology, 33,* 307–316.

Hogan, R. (1975). Empathy: A conceptual and psychometric analysis. *The Counseling Psychologist, 5*(2), 14–18.

Iannotti, R. J. (1975). The nature and measurement of empathy in children. *The Counseling Psychologist, 5*(2), 21–25.

Joel, L. A., & Collins, D. I. (1978). *Psychiatric nursing: theory and application.* New York: McGraw-Hill.

Kalisch, B. J. (1971). An experiment in the development of empathy in nursing students. *Nursing Research, 20,* 202–211.

Kerr, W. A. (1960). Diplomacy Test of Empathy. In R. S. Andrulis (Ed.), (1977), *Adult assessment: A source book of tests and measures of human behavior* (pp. 185–187). Springfield, IL: Charles C. Thomas.

Kunst-Wilson, W., Carpenter, L., Poser, A., Venohr, I., & Kushner, K. (1981). Empathic perceptions of nursing students: Self-reported and actual ability. *Research in Nursing and Health, 4,* 283–293.

La Monica, E. L. (1981). Construct validity of an empathy instrument. *Research in Nursing and Health, 4,* 389–400.

La Monica, E. L., Wolf, R. M., Madea, A. R., & Oberst, M. T. (1987). Empathy and nursing outcomes. *Scholarly Inquiry for Nursing Practice: An International Journal, 1,* 197–213.

Mehrabian, A., & Epstein, N. (1972). A measure of emotional empathy. *Journal of Personality, 40,* 525–543.

Namie, G. M. (1982/1983). Empathic and egoistic motivational bases of helping. From *Dissertation Abstracts International,* 1983, *43,* Abstract 2745B.

Orlando, I. J. (1972). *The discipline and teaching of nursing process*. New York: G. P. Putnam.

Orlando, I. J. (1961). *The dynamic nurse–patient relationship*. New York: G. P. Putnam.

Peitchinis, J. A. (1976). *Staff–patient communication in the health services*. New York: Springer Publishing Company.

Peplau, H. E. (1952). *Interpersonal relations in nursing: A conceptual frame of reference for psychodynamic nursing*. New York: G. P. Putnam.

Rogers, C. R. (1975). Empathic: An unappreciated way of being. *The Counseling Psychologist, 5*(2), 2–10.

Steibe, S. C., Boulet, D. B., & Lee, D. C. (1979). Trainee trait empathy, age, trainer functioning, client age and training time as discriminators of successful empathy training. *Canadian Counsellor, 14*(1), 41–46.

Stotland, E., Mathews, K. E., Jr., Sherman, S. E., Hansson, R. O., & Richardson, B. Z. (1978). *Empathy, fantasy, and helping*. Beverly Hills: Sage.

Szalita, A. B. (1976). Some thoughts on empathy. *Psychiatry, 39*, 142–152.

Toi, M., & Batson, C. D. (1982). More evidence that empathy is a source of altruistic motivation. *Journal of Personality and Social Psychology, 43*, 281–292.

Travelbee, J. (1966). *Interpersonal aspects of nursing*. Philadelphia: F. A. Davis.

Valle, S. K. (1981). Interpersonal functioning of alcoholism counselors and treatment outcome. *Journal of Studies on Alcohol, 42*, 783–790.

Wolf, F. M., Woolliscroft, J. O., Calhoun, J. G., & Boxer, G. J. (1987). A controlled experiment in teaching students to respond to patients' emotional concerns. *Journal of Medical Education, 62*, 25–34.

2

The Significance of Empathy

E. Joyce Carver
Jean R. Hughes

This chapter considers the significance of empathy first from a global perspective in relation to the major trends and issues within the health care system, and then in terms of health care team and patient–professional relationships. The proliferation of technology in the health care environment calls for empathic skills to humanize care. Changes in health–illness patterns require empathy as a crucial element in the management of chronic and terminal illness. The rise of consumerism challenges professionals to perceive citizen views empathically. Health professionals work as a team and should use empathy with each other to achieve less stressed, more productive collegial relationships. Active participation of patients in their health care demands empathy in each phase of problem solving within the professional–patient relationship.

The definition of empathy subscribed to here, and used in the empathy research reported later in this text, is that of La Monica (1981):

> Empathy signifies a central focus and feeling *with* and *in* the client's world. It involves accurate perception of the client's world by the helper, communication of this understanding to the client, and the client's perception of the helper's understanding (p. 398).

In this context empathy is not only a "way of being" with another (Rogers, 1975) but it also communicates to patients the professional's understanding of their world so that this perception can be validated by the patient. As Egan (1986) notes:

> It's the helper's way of saying, "I'm with you, I've been listening carefully to what you've been saying and expressing, and I'm checking to see if my understanding is accurate" (p. 99).

The significance of empathy is considered now in terms of the major trends and issues within the health care system.

CHANGING HEALTH CARE DEMANDS

Three distinct, ongoing changes in health care demands make the use of empathy skills increasingly important: the use of sophisticated technology, different health–illness patterns, and the rise of consumerism. These changes place increasing emphasis on the need for psychosocial care of patients accomplished through a helping relationship in which empathy is a basic ingredient. Next, each change will be addressed.

Increased Technology

Empathy is a high touch skill in a health care system dominated by large, impersonal institutions which rely on highly specialized diagnostic and treatment regimes using the latest equipment. The widespread growth of computers in many areas of patient care continues. Records and laboratory reports are automated and computerized in many institutions. Diagnostic tests, including images of internal body structures such as ultrasound, use computer technology. Advances continue in mechanical monitoring methods providing prompt and accurate physiologic information (Bronzino, 1982; Simpson & Brown, 1985). Howard (1975, p. 61) states that technology dehumanizes health care to such an extent that acute care patients may be viewed as extensions of machines. This phenomenon exists in many patient care situations.

The impersonal nature of a technical environment can produce obstacles to interpersonal openness and communication. This led Brunt (1985) to study nurses' empathy in the highly technical environment of the intensive care unit. He compared the ability of those nurses to that of nurses working in other areas of the hospital and found both groups to be non-facilitative and not significantly different in their use of empathy. Brunt recommended that empathy training be included in inservice and nursing school programs to increase empathy skills.

The sterility of a mechanical environment makes the caring, comforting functions of professionals critically important, yet difficult to achieve (Henderson, 1985). Technical competence is necessary, but must be combined with interpersonal skills such as empathy, warmth, and respect, before the patient feels health professionals' care (Purtilo & Cassel, 1981, p. 41). The proliferation of technology in health care means that patients require a sense of human caring and connectedness as never before. Technical care without professional caring is unlikely to satisfy patient needs, and may nullify the benefits of technology for patients concerned with the quality of life. Empathy provides a human bond which serves as a bridge to connect the patient to the social environment and helps to prevent a sense of isolation, alienation and loneliness (Northouse & Northouse, 1985; Smith, 1986).

Howard (1975) interviewed patients in several settings to determine the conditions necessary for humanized interaction in health care. Analysis of the interviews, observations of health facilities and the literature on personalization of care led Howard to identify empathy as a necessary variable for humanizing health care. Empathy helps professionals respond to patients as unique human beings because they can see the world from the vantage point of their patients and better understand their patients' needs (p. 83).

The increased use of technology presents patients, their families, and health care professionals, with overwhelmingly complex decisions/dilemmas which have many legal and ethical implications. For example, often decisions must be made about resuscitation of the terminally ill, organ transplants in the elderly, chemotherapy or radiation treatment for those with cancer, diagnostic tests or surgery which may involve considerable risks as well as cost, and the overall allocation of resources when the need exceeds the supply (Friedman Ed., 1986; Henderson, 1985). Patients are often afraid of invasive technical procedures and concerned about the quality of life extended only by machinery. Helping patients sort out their feelings, views and values is a necessary first step in making critical decisions, often with life-threatening outcomes.

Changing Patterns of Health–Illness

Many of the kinds of patient problems and requests health professionals face are shifting dramatically. As discussed below, aging of the population, increased life expectancy, and changes in the causes of illness and death are the major reasons for this.

The size of the older population is growing rapidly. The number of Canadians over 65 years of age has tripled in the last 55 years and is expected to triple in the next 45 years, with a significant growth in the number of those over 75 years of age and in the group aged 85 and over (Stone & Fletcher, 1986). For the first time in its history the United States has as many people aged 65 or over as teenagers (Schick, 1986). This trend is expected to continue with the proportion of the United States population 65 years and over increasing about 50 percent by the year 2020 (National Institute on Aging, 1987). The growth of the elderly population is even greater in Asia and European countries, while in some developing countries the over-60 age group is increasing faster than the total population (WHO, 1987). Lopez (1984) states that the increase in the elderly population of Europe will have the most impact on future health and social service requirements. Likewise, Rabin (1985) reports that the increase in the "old, old" of the United States is the most significant population change there.

Aside from a fall in the birth rate, the main reason for an aging population is increased life expectancy owing to lower infant mortality and decreased deaths from infectious diseases, the leading cause of death at the turn of the century (National Center for Health Statistics, 1988; Statistics Canada, 1985). Chronic diseases related to degenerative processes, more prevalent in the elderly, are now the leading cause of illness, disability and death. Cardiovascular diseases and cancer cause the greatest number of deaths in adults (National Center for Health Statistics, 1988; Statistics Canada, 1985; World Health Organization, 1987).

The illnesses and disabilities people live with place great demands on the health care system. The leading causes of hospitalization are heart disease, mental disorder, stroke, accidents and respiratory disease. Lifestyle factors over which people can assume some control, such as exercise, smoking, alcohol and drug use, eating habits and environmental stress, contribute to most of these illnesses. Mobility problems, such as arthritis, rheumatism and disease of the limbs and joints, account for two-thirds of all disability.

The highest incidence of disability is in the over-65 age group (Committee on an Aging Society, 1985; Statistics Canada, 1986; World Health Organization, 1987).

Helping the chronically ill modify and manage their living situation requires caring because major emotional adjustments must be addressed (World Health Organization, 1987, p. 12). Extensive lifestyle alterations often have to be made (Heikkinen, 1987). New knowledge and skills about treatment and control must be learned. Cure is usually not possible. Traditionally, the health care system has focused on curing illnesses which call for the high technology of hospitals. LaLonde (1974) advocates a shift from curing to caring. He notes that the caring function is not as satisfying as curing because treatment of chronic illness is not as dramatic and success cannot easily be measured. He believes that the value system of health care organizations has to change from cure of acute illness to care for the chronically ill. Care will need to become as rewarding for professionals as the cure of acute conditions. Empathy is a part of that caring.

As the age of the population increases, and along with it the number of chronic and debilitating illnesses, care of those in nursing and residential homes deserves more attention. Williams (1979) studied the effects of empathy in the nursing care of the institutionalized aged to determine if empathy might offset the dehumanization and depersonalization of the person's environment as measured by changes in self-concept. Nurse therapists offered low and high level empathy to groups of elderly institutionalized individuals over an 8-week period. There was a statistically significant increase in the self-concept of subjects in the groups with the nurse therapist offering high versus low empathy responses. The study concluded that the level of empathy used ". . . has a strong probability of enhancing or depreciating the self-concept of the institutionalized aged" (p. 24).

The mental health needs of the population clearly demand empathic professionals. Statistics on mental disorders are very inadequate because many people do not seek treatment owing to the shame or fear still associated with mental illness (Searl, Hughes, & Majumdar, 1985, p. 133). As well, unreported emotional distress and anxiety are frequent reasons for seeking general medical care and often occur in relation to other illnesses or absenteeism from work. Reported cases, mainly those hospitalized, account only for the most severely ill.

Nevertheless, hospitalization for mental disorders accounts for slightly more than 8 percent of all patient days in both mental institutions and general hospitals (Statistics Canada, 1985). Vital statistics for the United States show an alarming increase in suicide rates in young adults, especially among white males (National Center for Health Statistics, 1988). Heikkinen (1987, p. 25) notes that the older population has a mean prevalence of about 25 percent for mental disorders. Blazer (1985) advocates the use of empathy in the care of those with late-life depression. Empathy is essential to the therapeutic relationship, the main instrument in the treatment of mental illness.

The current epidemic of Acquired Immune Deficiency Syndrome (AIDS) requires great interpersonal skill in the psychosocial care of its victims and their families (Haines, 1987; National Institute of Mental Health, 1986). Both care and prevention require highly developed empathic skills to understand the feelings and meet the needs of those served. Health professionals have the arduous task of conveying emotionally charged information to the public concerning such diseases as AIDS. Fear, anger, and misconceptions lead some to believe in discriminatory practices. In the midst of such fear, health professionals themselves may be ostracized by family and friends because they care for patients with socially undesirable diseases.

Helping patients cope with terminal illness and enabling them to die peacefully in a manner and location of their choice requires listening to and understanding of patient needs. Hospice units, hospice care workers, and hospice volunteer programs have mushroomed (Ellerton & Downe-Wamboldt, 1987; Mahar, 1981). The hospice concept developed because of deficient psychosocial care in acute care institutions (Mahar, 1981, p. 370; Osterweis, Solomon, & Green, 1984, p. 215). Hospice care activities feature empathy skills in the provision of emotional support to dying patients, their families, and close friends.

Family violence is now a major health and social issue. The real extent of problems owing to child abuse, wife battering, and abuse of the elderly is just becoming publicly known (Duggan, 1981; Foley & Grimes, 1987). The root causes include an absence of healthy interpersonal relationships, which must be the prime focus of empathic care and prevention. The incidence of family violence may be viewed as a barometer of the need for relationship skills in our society as a whole. Aspy (1975, p. 13) suggests that the benefit of empathic interactions extends beyond the health care system to the entire society and that empathy training should be available for everyone.

Empathy plays a vital role in the therapy advocated for family violence. Group self-help approaches recommended by Petit (1981, p. 291) and Valenti (1986, p. 132) require empathic skills to encourage sharing and to allow the group to take primary responsibility for bringing about change. Valenti states that an important part of the helping process with abused women is the professional's ability to discover how women see their problems and their readiness to change. Empathy provides professionals with a glimpse of the world in which abused people live.

The above changes in health–illness patterns place greater demands on the ability of health professionals to understand and effectively work with patients' emotional reactions and feelings about their altered life situation. They underscore the need to focus more energies on the prevention and management of illness outside of hospitals. The need for counseling and public education about lifestyle, personal decision making, and self-responsibility for health is becoming more obvious. The move from curing to caring demands empathic skills that involve the patient as an active participant in the helping relationship.

Consumerism

Consumer organizations now exert considerable influence on the health care system and cannot be ignored. There is growing dissatisfaction about the quality and delivery of health care. Citizens are demanding a voice in the decision-making process about their own health care and about the planning of health programs (Gordon, 1981; Hamilton, 1982; Storch, 1982).

The consumer movement represents a change in how the public views the expertise and authority of health care providers. The elitist role traditionally assumed by professionals is no longer tolerated (Curtin & Flaherty, 1982, p. 81). Consumers are forcing health professionals to work jointly with them and are insisting that citizens play an active role in health care decisions (Gordon, 1981).

Rising costs have helped to stimulate the development of greater consumer participation in health care matters. The public wants a say in how their health care dollars will be spent. The ability of modern medicine to extend life seems almost endless, but the resources to do so are limited. Difficult decisions must be made about who will be treated and who may be allowed to die. Public trust in the ability of health care providers to make these decisions is waning (Storch, 1982).

Most consumer complaints about health care identify a lack of individualized, human contact rather than inadequate physical care (Clausen, 1979; Gazda, 1975, p. 1; Fisher, 1981). Many believe that the bureaucratization of hospitals and health care organizations is a cause of impersonal, dehumanized care (Storch, 1982, p. 6; Aiken & Aiken, 1973). Empathy skills help ensure that patients are viewed as individuals by professionals who are sensitive to their views.

The self-help movement is further evidence of consumer disenchantment with the quality of care related to our need for human sharing and understanding. The proliferation of self-help groups is a world-wide phenomenon of such strength that it has been called a revolution (Gartner & Riessman Eds., 1984). Others believe it symbolizes the need for a fundamental reorientation in the provision of health care which would allow patients a more active role in problem-solving, especially concerning their needs for practical and emotional support (Kickbusch & Hatch, 1983, p. 1). Self-help groups exist for all ages and address an increasing variety of diseases and psychosocial problems. They represent a significant force in augmenting the ability of individuals to take charge of their own lives. It appears that these groups fill a void in health and social care: empathic listening and understanding.

Health professionals face the challenge of working with self-help groups in a collaborative relationship which emphasizes equality. Unfortunately professionals tend not to support self-help groups perhaps because they cannot relate to groups over which they do not exercise control. Romeder (1982, p. 90) believes this constitutes a major opposing force to self-help groups. Professionals must learn to work in a more equal partnership with lay people and to respect patients' inherent ability to take action on their own problems. Empathic understanding forms a basis for this approach (see Gazda & Evans, Chapter 5 of this text). Self-help groups provide human support and caring which professionals often cannot provide. Participants have experienced the problems faced by those in the group and therefore can identify with each other's frames of reference. Empathy is the main tool by which professionals without such personal experience gain an understanding of the patient's world.

Patient rights are an issue in health care consumerism (Hamilton, 1982; Storch, 1982). Effective relationship skills ensure that a number of patient rights are met: the right to be respected; the right to participate, and the right to be informed. Failure to recognize these rights leads to patient grievances and legal action. The increase in malpractice suits indicates that personal relationships deteriorate frequently or that they often do not develop. Rozovsky (1980, p. 128) believes improved human relationships between patients and health care providers will help prevent legal action. Empathy is a key to satisfactory relationships.

EMPATHY WITHIN THE HEALTH CARE TEAM

Health professionals work in teams involving colleagues from a wide variety of disciplines, such as social workers, physicians, clergy, nurses, nutritionists, pharmacists, and physical therapists, to name only a few. Effective team functioning requires that each member understand the role and perspective of other members. Conflict within the health care team often results from lack of understanding and poor communication about what should be done, by whom, and when (Northouse & Northouse, 1985, p. 100; Smith, 1986, p. 285). Empathy enables each team member to understand the pressures faced by the others, to respect the beliefs held by those in different disciplines, and to appreciate the realm of patient care each handles most effectively (Northouse & Northouse, 1985, p. 36). In recognition of this, Anderson & Gerrard (1984) include empathy skills as an important focus in their educational program which prepares nurses to handle common interpersonal problems, including team conflict. Empathic understanding contributes to effective team functioning, professional satisfaction, and better patient care. Gazda, Walters & Childers (1975) state:

> "If more care, concern, respect and understanding is communicated between health care professionals, less anxiety and frustration will arise. If these qualities are communicated to persons receiving health care, there will be less fear and dissatisfaction, more trust in the professional and paraprofessional helper, and greater benefits will accrue to the giver and the receiver of health care." (p. 2)

Empathy plays a role in other aspects of collegial communication. Kramer and Schmalenberg (1977) believe it can help resolve

the conflicts which arise during the adjustments of newly graduated professionals to the work world. They studied the conflicts
faced by nurses in their first job resulting from competing values
and expectations of the two subcultures: professional versus bureaucratic. For example, the school subculture may place emphasis
on individualized patient care while the work subculture is more
concerned about the organization of and care for all patients. Kramer and Schmalenberg state that the resolution of these conflicts
requires both old and new staff to develop biculturalism, that is, to
become comfortable functioning with the values and expectations
of both school and work settings. They write that empathy plays a
crucial role in the ability to become bicultural because it enables co-
workers to understand and accurately anticipate the thoughts, feelings and actions of the other (p. 13). They elaborate further on the
need for those in administration to understand the adjustments of
new graduates and use this time as a basis for empathy development between new graduates and other staff. Gazda, Childers, &
Walters (1982, p. 232) concur that empathy is important in
supervisor–employee communication because empathy enables the
supervisor to understand the employee's goals and needs.

Empathy provided by one member of the health team to another
can help professionals cope with the rigorous and constant demands faced in their work and help prevent burnout. Hazardous
stress levels can be relieved by professionals who are responsive to
the emotional needs of their co-workers and encourage them to
express their feelings (McConnell, 1982; Jones, 1982; Mullins, &
Barstow, 1982). The inclusion of empathic interchanges in peer
support groups and staff meetings serves this purpose (Valenti,
1986, p. 133; Pines, Aronson, & Kafry, 1981, p. 134). Colleagues
who are in emotional distress can benefit from the same empathic
skills used with patients. Smith (1986) examines such situations
and suggests strategies using empathy for communicating with
colleagues who are upset, sad, or depressed. Cohen & McQuade
(1983) agree with this approach and have prepared a unit of pro-
grammed instruction on developing empathy with co-workers using situations involving nurses and other professionals in hospital
settings.

Empathy is important in professional–professional relationships
both in team and one-to-one situations. The need to use empathy
is not restricted to any one level of care giver. Empathy should be
used by co-workers, novices, veterans, managers, and educators
alike.

PROFESSIONAL–PATIENT RELATIONSHIPS

The ultimate goal of professional–patient relationships is patient action to resolve a problem and enhance the patient's level of functioning. Empathy is an important skill in each step of the problem-solving cycle as explained by Gazda and Evans in Chapter 5 of this book.

The significance of empathy within the professional–patient relationship revolves around a certain view of the patient's role in that relationship: that patients have the resources and integrity to play an active role in solving their problems. Operating from this framework, the professional plays a facilitative rather than a controlling role and resists the natural tendency to make decisions for the patient.

The effects of empathy on the quality of patient care is the focus of several chapters in this book. Research shows a positive relationship between professional empathy and outcome. Aspy (1975) and Rogers (1975) summarize studies which conclude that empathy is related to the positive outcomes of patient self-exploration, learning and change in psychotherapy, and learning in the classroom. Referring to Rogers (1975), Gladstein (1977) believes empathy may be more helpful when a person is hurting, confused, troubled, or anxious. Subsequent chapters of this book specifically address the relationship of empathy and patient well-being.

SUMMARY

Empathy provides a "high touch" skill in a "high tech" health care world; an environment in which health professionals need to use empathy to humanize their interactions with each other as well as with their patients. Health–illness patterns are transforming the reasons many patients seek health care. The swing is towards older patients with chronic or terminal illnesses which urgently need caring. Spurred on by concerns about the cost and quality of health care, consumers are demanding a more active role in decisions regarding their own health and the formation of policy for society as a whole. They are challenging health professionals to understand consumer beliefs and concerns. Critical to this understanding is the dimension of empathy. The following chapters explore how professionals learn to use empathy and the effect of professional empathy on patient well-being.

REFERENCES

Aiken, L., & Aiken, J. (1973). A systematic approach to the evaluation of interpersonal relationships. *American Journal of Nursing, 73*(4), 863–867.

Anderson, H., & Gerrard, B. (1984). A comprehensive interpersonal skills program for nurses. *Journal of Nursing Education, 23*(8), 353–355.

Aspy, D. N. (1975). Empathy: Let's get the hell on with it. *The Counseling Psychologist, 5*(2), 10–14.

Blazer, D. (1984). Depressive illness in late life. In Committee on an Aging Society. *America's aging: Health in an older society* (pp. 105–128). Washington, D.C.: National Academy Press.

Bronzino, J. D. (1982). *Computer applications for patient care.* Reading, MA: Addison-Wesley.

Brunt, J. H. (1985). An exploration of the relationship between nurses' empathy and technology. *Nursing Administration Quarterly, 9*(4), 69–78.

Clausen, J. P. (1979). Humanizing health care. In D. Hymovich, & M. W. Barnard, (Eds.). *Family health care* (Vol. 11, 2nd ed.). pp. 235–242. New York: McGraw-Hill.

Cohen, S., & McQuade, K. (1983). Developing empathy with co-workers. *American Journal of Nursing, 83*(2), 1573–1588.

Committee on an Aging Society (1985). *America's aging: Health in an older society.* Washington, D.C.: National Academy Press.

Curtin, L., & Flaherty, M. J. *Nursing ethics: Theories and pragmatics.* Bowie, MD: Robert J. Brady.

Duggan, M. (1981). Violence in the family. In C. Getty, & W. Humphreys, (Eds.). *Understanding the family: Stress and change in American family life.* (pp. 253–270). New York: Appleton-Century-Crofts.

Egan, G. (1986). *The skilled helper: A systematic approach to effective helping.* (3rd ed.). Monterey, CA: Brooks/Cale.

Ellerton, M., & Downe-Wamboldt, B. (1987). The concerns of hospice patients and the role of hospice volunteers. *Journal of Palliative Care, 3*(1), 16–22.

Fisher, J. (1981). A continuing education workshop on human relations skills. *Nursing Papers, 13*(3), 27–36.

Foley, T. S., & Grimes, B. A. (1987). Nursing intervention in family abuse and violence. In G. W. Stuart, & S. J. Sundeen, (Eds.), *Principles and Practice of Psychiatric Nursing* (3rd ed.) (pp. 926–970). St. Louis, MO: C. V. Mosby Co.

Friedman, E. (Ed.). (1986). *Making choices: Ethics issues for health care professionals.* Baskerville: American Hospital Publishing Inc.

Gartner, A., & Riessman, F. (Eds.). (1984). *The Self-Help Revolution* (Vol. X). New York: Human Sciences Press.

Gazda, G. M., Walters, R. P., & Childers, W. C. (1975). *Human relations development: A manual for health sciences.* Boston, MA: Allyn and Bacon.

Gazda, G. M., Childers, W. C., & Walters, R. P. (1982). *Interpersonal com-*

munication: A handbook for health professionals. Rockville, MD: Aspen Publishers.

Gladstein, G. A. (1977). Empathy and counseling outcome: An empirical and conceptual review. *The Counseling Psychologist, 6*(4), 70–79.

Gordon, I. T. (1981). Inroads in consumer participation. *The Canadian Nurse, 77*(8), 38–42.

Haines, J. (1987). AIDS: New considerations in caring. *The Canadian Nurse, 83*(1), p. 11–12.

Hamilton, P. A. (1982). *Health care consumerism.* St. Louis: C. V. Mosby.

Heikkinen, E. (1987). Health implications of population aging in Europe. *World Health Statistics Quarterly, 40*(1), 22–40.

Henderson, V. (1985). The essence of nursing in high technology. *Nursing Administration Quarterly, 9*(4) 1–9

Howard, J. (1975). Humanization and dehumanization of health care. In J. Howard & A. Strauss (Eds.), *Humanizing health care,* (pp. 57–102). New York: John Wiley.

Jones, E. M. (1982). Who supports the nurse? In E. McConnell (Ed.), *Burnout in the nursing profession: Coping strategies, causes and costs.* (pp. 246–249). St. Louis, MO: C.V. Mosby.

Kickbusch, I., & Hatch, S. (1983). A re-orientation of health care? In S. Hatch, & I. Kickbusch (Eds.), *Self-help and health in Europe: New approaches in health care,* (pp. 1–9). Copenhagen: World Health Organization.

Kramer, M., & Schmalenberg, C. (1977). The first job . . . a proving ground: Basis for empathy development. *Journal of Nursing Administration, 7*(1), 12–20.

LaLonde, M. (1974). *A new perspective in the health of Canadians.* Ottawa: Government of Canada.

La Monica, E. L. (1981). Construct validity of an empathic instrument. *Research in Nursing and Health, 4,* 389–400.

Lopez, A. D. (1984). Demographic change in Europe and its health and social implications: An overview. In A. D. Lopez & R. L. Cliquet (Eds.), *Demographic trends in the European Region* (pp. 5–67). Copenhagen: World Health Organization Regional Publications, European Series No. 17.

Mahar, I. (1981). The hospice concept: An alternative approach to terminal care. In C. Getty, & W. Humphreys (Eds.), *Understanding the family: Stress and change in American family life,* (pp. 370–381). New York: Appleton-Century-Crofts.

McConnell, E. A. (1982). Coping strategies for preventing burnout. In E. A. McConnell (Ed.), *Burnout in the nursing profession: Coping strategies, causes and costs,* (pp. 1–8) St. Louis, MO.: C. V. Mosby.

Mullins, A. C., & Barstow, R. E. (1982). Care for the caretakers. In E. McConnell (Ed.), *Burnout in the nursing profession: Coping strategies, causes and costs.* (pp. 53–56). St. Louis, MO.: C. V. Mosby.

National Center for Health Statistics (1988). *Health United States 1987.* (DHHS Publication No. PHS 88–1232). Washington, D.C.: U. S. Government Printing Office.

National Institute of Mental Health. (1986). *Coping with AIDS: Psychological and social considerations in helping people with HTV-III infection.* (DHHS Publication No. ADM 85–1432). Washington, DC. U.S. Government Printing Office.

National Institution on Aging. (1987). *Personnel for health needs of the elderly through the year 2020.* (NIH Publication No. 87-2950). Bethesda, MD: National Institutes of Health.

Northouse, P. B., & Northouse, L. L. (1985). *Health communication: A Handbook for health professionals.* Englewood Cliffs, NJ: Prentice-Hall.

Osterweis, M., Solomon, F., & Green, M. (Eds.). (1984). *Bereavement: Reactions, consequences, and care.* Washington, D.C.: National Academy Press.

Petit, M. (1981). Battered women: A (nearly) hidden social problem. In C. Getty & W. Humphreys (Eds.), *Understanding the family: Stress and change in American family life,* (pp. 272–297). New York: Appleton-Century-Crofts.

Pines, A. M., Aronson, E., & Kafry, D. (1981). *Burnout: From tedium to personal growth.* New York: The Free Press.

Purtilo, R. B., & Cassel, C. K. (1981). *Ethical dimensions in the health professions.* Philadelphia: W. B. Saunders.

Rabin, D. L. (1985). Waxing of the gray, waning of the green. In Committee on an Aging Society. *America's aging: Health in an older society* (pp. 28–56). Washington, D.C.: National Academy Press.

Rogers, C. R. (1975). Empathic: An unappreciated way of being. *The Counseling Psychologist,* 5, 2–10.

Romeder, J. (1982). *Self-help groups in Canada.* Ottawa: Health and Welfare Canada.

Rozovsky, L. E. (1980). *The Canadian patients' book of rights.* Toronto: Doubleday Canada.

Schick, F. L. (Ed.). (1986). *Statistical handbook on aging Americans.* Phoenix, AZ: Oryx Press.

Searl, S., Hughes, J., & Majumdar, B. (1985). The health status of Canadians. In M. Stewart, J. Innis, S. Searl & C. Smillie (Eds.). *Community health nursing in Canada.* (pp. 129–141). Toronto: Gage Educational.

Simpson, R. L., & Brown, L. N. (1985). High-touch/high-technology computer applications in nursing. *Nursing Administration Quarterly,* 9(4), 62–68.

Smith, S. (1986). *Communications in nursing: Communicating assertively and responsibly in nursing.* Toronto: McGraw-Hill Ryerson.

Statistics Canada (1985). *Canada Year Book 1985.* Ottawa: Statistics Canada.

Statistics Canada (1986). *Report of the Canadian health and disability survey.* Ottawa: Statistics Canada.

Stone, L. O., & Fletcher, S. (1986). *The seniors boom: Dramatic increases in longevity and prospects for better health.* Ottawa: Statistics Canada.

Storch, J. (1982). *Patients' rights: Ethical and legal issues in health care and nursing.* Toronto: McGraw-Hill Ryerson.

Valenti, C. (1986). Working with the physically abused woman. In D. K. Kjervick & I. M. Martinson (Eds.), *Women in health and illness: Life experience and crises.* (pp. 127–133). Philadelphia: W. B. Saunders.

Williams, C. L. (1979). Empathic communication and its effect on client outcome. *Issues in Mental Health Nursing.* 2(1), 15–26.

World Health Organization. (1987). *World health statistics annual.* Geneva: WHO.

3

The Historical Roots of Empathy in the Helping Professions

Jacquelyn Peitchinis

This chapter presents some history in the development of the concept of empathy from its linguistic roots in ancient times to its present theorists' concerns. It does not attempt to be comprehensive, but rather to provide some indication of the nature of its development over the years. From the ideas of a German psychologist in the latter part of the nineteenth century, the notion of empathy has grown to be considered a factor in human relations. Much could be written in relation to its developing use by workers in the health and social services, but this will be limited for the most part to some influences on the nursing and health professions.

Concepts vaguely related to empathy have a long history in human experience and language (Barrett-Lennard, 1981, p. 91). Evidently *empatheia* was an early Greek word meaning affection and passion with a quality of suffering (Ibid.) Barrett-Lennard (1981) points out that "the *em* means "in" or "into" and there is the idea at least of going into a strong feeling/connection with another" (p. 91). The Latin equivalent, largely borrowed from the Greek, was *pathos* which can mean feeling/perception (Ibid.).

EINFÜHLUNG—EMPATHY

The word empathy was introduced by Edward B. Titchener, an English psychologist at Cornell University, in the early part of this century, to be the English equivalent of the German word, *Einfüh-lung*. The latter term was coined about 1885 by Theodor Lipps, a German psychologist, to mean the aesthetic experience related to contemplation of plastic arts, such as sculpture (Szalita, 1976). Ein-fühlung literally means "feeling into." For Lipps, an aesthetic object represented a living being: projection of myself into the object's life bringing about a specific psychic state. Szalita (1976) considered Freud's essay on Michelangelo's statue of Moses in Rome to be a good illustration of Lipps' view of Einfühlung. Freud drew inferences not only from the statue but also from his personal inner response to it and developed a hypothesis about Michelangelo's intention.

Lipps thought that empathy gave the most satisfactory account of individuals' knowledge of others (Allport, 1937, p. 531). Quoting from Lipps' 1903 writings, Allport states: "There are three spheres of knowledge. I know about things, about myself, and about others. . . . The source of the third type of knowledge is empathy (Einfühlung)" (1937, p. 531n). By coining the term *empathy*, Titchener introduced American readers to Lipps' concepts. (Stotland et al., 1978, pp. 11–12). Psychologist William McDougall used the word empathy in 1908 to mean "a primitive process of emotional contagion" (Stotland et al., 1978, p. 12). McDougall thought that empathy may or may not lead to helping behavior. (Gladstein, 1983, p. 474).

EMPATHY IN PSYCHOANALYSIS

Freud acknowledged the term empathy. One notes in a revision of a 1921 text that he stated:

> . . . we are faced by the process which psychology calls "empathy" [Einfühlung] and which plays the largest part in our understanding of what is inherently foreign to our ego in other people (1967, p. 40).

Freud also wrote: "A path leads from identification by way of imitation to empathy, that is, to the comprehension of the mechanism by means of which we are enabled to take up any attitude at all towards another mental life" (1967, p. 42n). Using as reference Jones' (1959) *Collected Papers of Sigmund Freud*, Khajavi and Hekmat (1971, p. 490) have stated that Freud indicated, "empathy serves a prime function in establishing rapport. . . ."

Among the pioneer psychoanalysts, Alfred Adler is considered to have recognized the importance of empathy in therapy. Adler reportedly stated, "We must be able to see with his eyes and listen with his ears" (Barrett-Lennard 1981, p. 92). Psychoanalysts talked at the end of the second decade of this century of oscillating and blending free associations, empathy, intuition, introspection, problem solving, thinking, theoretical knowledge and other techniques (Greenson, 1967, p. 100). The analyst was to be empathic with the patient's emotional life but retain his dispassionate understanding (Ibid., p. 279). For Greenson (1967) the psychoanalyst, empathy meant "to share, to experience the feelings of another human being" (p. 368).

Greenson (1967) cites a source as early as 1941 in stating that if the psychoanalyst is to be scientific, he must oscillate between using empathy and intuition and using his theoretical knowledge (p. 16). According to Greenson, empathy "is essential for psychological-mindedness and is dependent on the capacity for temporary and partial identification with others" (p. 54). For Stewart (1956), who based his concept of empathy on Freud's ideas, empathy involves deliberate identification. Empathy is

> . . . both a process of intuition and the basis of dynamic inference. . . . Empathy . . . is not just a putting oneself in the other's place as one casually *sees* the other, or as one is infected by a stray emotional feeling. Effort and imagination, choice and deliberation, and therefore creative selection are required by the empathic act (pp. 12–13).

There is a psychological distance between two people in empathy according to Stewart. Each has his own identity and is conscious of it. Neither is possessed or overpowered "by outside influences as in crude identification" (p. 14).

Truax and Carkhuff (1967, p. 39) have maintained that empathy "has long been a central tool in psychoanalysis." Quoting from psychoanalyst Fliess' writings of 1942, Katz (1963, p. 13) has stated that the skill of the therapist depends

> . . . essentially on his ability to put himself in the latter's place, to step into his shoes, and to obtain in this way an inside knowledge that is almost first-hand. The common name for such a procedure is "empathy"; and we, as a suitable name for it in our nomenclature, should like to suggest calling it trial identification.

The concept of empathy was adopted in various human relations situations for good or otherwise. Some considered it a "hidden persuader" (Szalita, 1976, p. 150). According to Szalita (1976), the German playwright Bertolt Brecht "repeatedly observing Hitler's manipulative use of empathy . . . became convinced that the theater had to be liberated from empathy and catharsis" (p. 150). In the 1950s a film shown in North America entitled *Funny Face* (Paramount, 1956) was an amusing satire on empathy—it ridiculed the concept.

PSYCHOTHERAPY AND COUNSELING

In 1940, Carl Rogers (1951, p. 9) presented the first paper outlining the principles and techniques of a new approach to psychotherapy which soon became known as "nondirective counseling." The paper was revised and published as the second chapter of Rogers' *Counseling and Psychotherapy* (1942). In this work Rogers did not use the term empathy, but through case excerpts drew attention to the counselor's clarification and acceptance of the client's feelings. Reporting on a comparison of directive and nondirective phonographically recorded interviews, Rogers revealed that the latter were almost ten times more likely to respond " . . . in such a way as to indicate recognition of expression of feeling or attitude in immediately preceding verbal response" (1942, p. 121). Three of the most frequently used techniques of nondirective counselors were recognizing in some way the feeling or attitude which the client had just expressed; interpreting or recognizing feelings or attitudes by general demeanor, specific behavior or earlier statements; and recognizing the subject content of what the client had just said (p. 123).

Empathy was having an impact in the field of social work. In

1946, Charlotte Towle wrote of the client–social worker relationship as being " . . . a warm relationship in which the worker feels into and with the client without feeling like him. . . . The worker affords the client a relatively neutral but understanding response" (Perlman, 1969, p. 104). In general it seems that counseling in social work has followed the psychoanalytic tradition. However, the desirability of this tradition has been questioned (Fischer, 1976).

THE MANY MEANINGS OF EMPATHY

It was 1949 when Rosalind Dymond drew attention to the many different meanings ascribed to empathy. She also referred to the fact that she developed the only test known purporting to measure empathy. Dymond viewed empathy as the ability to take the role of another. She commented that "some of us are highly sensitive and perceptive of what the other fellow is thinking and how he is feeling, while others are very obtuse and slow about picking up these clues" (p. 133). She wondered why, and if one could be trained to be empathic. In a subsequent study, Dymond (1950) found that high empathizers were outgoing, optimistic, warm, emotional people with a strong interest in others (p. 349). Low empathizers were, among other things, rather rigid, introverted and subject to uncontrolled emotionality.

Nondirective counseling developed into client-centered therapy, an approach to human relations, in the decade following Carl Rogers' initial (1940) paper (Rogers, 1951, p. 12). Empathy was an important ingredient in client-centered therapy. In Rogers' words:

> . . . it is the counselor's function to assume, in so far as he is able, the internal frame of reference of the client, to perceive the world as the client sees it, to perceive the client himself as he is seen by himself, to lay aside all perceptions from the external frame of reference while doing so, and to communicate something of this empathic understanding to the client (1951, p. 29).

Rogers pointed out that empathy is not an emotional identification. The counselor perceives the client's hopes, hates and fears but does not experience them (p. 29).

In the nursing literature it is noted that Peplau, a nursing teacher at Columbia University, had two references to empathy in her 1952 book, *Interpersonal Relations in Nursing*. This was the same year Eysenck (1952) concluded from a study of the relevant literature that beneficial effects of psychotherapy were not proven. An outcome of Eysenck's criticism was an increase in research on the effectiveness of therapy which attempted to employ more sophisticated research designs. In 1954, Rogers and Dymond reported on more than four years' progress in an ongoing research program in psychotherapy at the Counseling Center of the University of Chicago. The research was concerned with process and outcomes of therapy in the client-centered or nondirective approach. Although Rogers and Dymond admitted that the research "contains a multitude of tantalizing unanswered questions" (p. 426), they concluded that the findings supported the theory of client-centered therapy (p. 433). Empathy was an important part of this theory.

EMPATHY AND HEALTH WORKERS

As has been indicated, the concept of empathy began to have some influence in nursing by the 1950s. Speroff wrote in 1956 that empathy was important in nursing. In the same year, Carl Rogers presented a paper to the Public Health Nurses' Section of the biennial convention of the American Nurses' Association in Chicago. The paper was adapted and published in *American Journal of Nursing* in August 1956. Rogers discussed the therapeutic relationship which included a "sensitive empathy" and hypothesized

> . . . that to the degree that the nurse can create such a relationship with her patient, she will release in the patient psychological strengths which promote growth and healing and which parallel the physiological forces operating in that direction (p. 997).

In 1958 Rogers published the Characteristics of a Helping Relationship in the *Personnel and Guidance Journal* (Rogers, 1962). He asks the question, "Can I let myself enter freely into the world of his feelings and personal meanings and see these as he does?" (p. 12–13).

By 1957 Rogers had published his "Necessary and Sufficient Conditions of Therapeutic Personality Change." One of these conditions was the therapist's experiencing "an empathic understanding of the client's internal frame of reference" and endeavoring to communicate this to the client (p. 96). For Rogers (1957) it was important "to sense the client's private world as if it were your own, but without ever losing the "as if" quality—this is empathy, and this seems essential to therapy" (p. 99).

Some fifteen years later two physicians described the ideal clinician as relating to his patient with empathy—"the ability to understand and appreciate how the patient feels without being distressed himself." (Engel & Morgan, Jr., 1973 p. 14). Before Rogers' (1957) aforementioned publication, Szasz and Hollender (1956) stated that the mutual participation model of physician–patient interaction was essentially foreign to medicine. Previous to this indictment, Dr. Brian Bird of Western Reserve University wrote a delightful little book, *Talking with Patients* (1955), in which he emphasized the importance of encouraging the patient to talk about himself and his problems and the necessity of the physician to listen intently if he is to help the patient. In a second edition in 1973, Bird wrote of the importance of listening to the person to determine what he actually thinks, feels, fears and desires (Preface p. vii).

In the 1960s the health and social services were being criticized in some measure for their lack of concern for the psychological care of their patients and suggestions were being made to them for addressing this issue. Ruesch (1961), a communication theorist, stated:

> The presence of another person who understands, acknowledges, and responds to the patient is a prerequisite for therapeutic communication. This person may be a doctor, nurse, relative or friend (p. 462).

Evang (1960), the Director General of Health Services in Norway, in a lecture at the University of London in 1958, maintained:

> . . . while we have tremendously developed the material, technical and scientific aspects of hospitals, we have not been able to fill the impressive frame with a corresponding amount of human understanding, warmth and appreciation of the strength of the human mind (p. 63).

Jourard (1961) wrote to a nursing audience, "Those who have become sick may be treated less with drugs and surgery, and more with human relations that heal" (p. 634). Bettelheim (1962) communicated to nurses the importance of seeing things from the patient's point of view—especially children's—and of the need to take time to talk to patients to know how they see their worlds.

Some nurses were attempting to develop a more therapeutic approach to nursing practice. In their book, *Science Principles Applied to Nursing*, Nordmark and Rohweder (1959) referred to the nurse's function of assisting the patient to communicate needs, desires and feelings and of indicating understanding and acceptance of these. Orlando offered a theory of effective nursing practice in 1961. Although she did not employ the term empathy it seems implied. The author pointed out the necessity for establishing a helpful relationship with patients to assist them to express the nature and meaning of their distress or need, and to ascertain the help required for relief. Nurses validated the accuracy of their perceptions and the helpfulness or appropriateness of their actions with the patient. Wiedenbach (1964) in her book, *Clinical Nursing: A Helping Act*, stated:

> The nurse's area of responsibility, although seldom specifically defined is, I think, *the patient's perception of his condition.* She has opportunity, by virtue of her close and continuous association with the patient, to detect how he is experiencing his condition or situation and why he experiences it as he does (p. 12).

Henderson (1964) has written of the nurse's requirement to know and understand the patient—to "get inside his skin" (p. 66).

Writing about the clinical psychiatric nurse in 1966, Holmes and Werner stated:

> It is helpful if she can let herself experience the world as the patient does, that is, actually experience to a limited extent the feelings the patient is having. This is empathy in the true sense . . . (p. 83).

In the same year Wilder Penfield, the internationally known Canadian neurosurgeon, wrote:

> I will let no patient leave my office or my laboratory, and I will pass no sick bed, until I have looked at life through the patient's eyes and made an effort to help in one way or another (p. 87).

In an introductory nursing text in 1967, Kozier and Du Gas stated the ability to empathize, "is to sense and appreciate how another person feels and to communicate this understanding to him" (p. 23). Writing about the nurse and her patient in 1968, Lockerby maintained that, ". . . unless the nurse knows what he wants, how he feels, what concerns him, she cannot fulfill her role" (p. 34). This writer thought that the nurse "must accept and fulfill the patient's expectations of her empathic role" (p. 5). It is to be noted that there were nurses who warned their colleagues against "unwarranted trust in the concept of empathy when helping those who are ill" (Peitchinis, 1976, p. 44). Later, in 1978, Hackney raised serious doubts about the effectiveness of empathy in counseling.

In the practice of medicine the family doctor probably had always been empathic. However in 1970, Taylor expressed the view that the family doctor had virtually disappeared and that the physician now diagnoses the disease, decides what to do about it, and maintains social distance between himself and the patient to establish his authority (pp. 165, 170). In 1974 Bates reported that studies demonstrate that "many physicians are more skilled and comfortable in meeting patients' needs for drugs and for diagnostic or therapeutic technologies than they are in providing a trusting relationship and skilled understanding" (p. 71). There is evidence that this is probably not so in many instances. The doctor–patient relationship has been described by physicians Witthower and Warnes (1977) as an alliance between an empathic doctor and a patient who is helped to help himself (p. 30). But as recently as 1982, Streit-Forest indicated that medical students were not learning to be empathic. At the same time Elizur and Rosenheim (1982) demonstrated that although medical students were more empathic than other science students, they were less so than those in the psychosocial disciplines. The same researchers found that group experience in a psychiatric clerkship could enhance medical students' ability to be empathic.

In the 1980s physicians and surgeons began writing more about the concept of empathy and its importance in physician–patient relations. In the view of a surgeon, communication with patients requires empathy defined as "putting yourself in the other person's shoes" (Calnan, 1983, p. 22). A physician has stated that to empathize with a patient "is to understand not only the factual implications of her words, but also the importance to her of what she is describing" (Cassell, 1985, p. 138).

FURTHER DEVELOPMENTS IN THE CONCEPT
OF EMPATHY

While health professionals were attempting to incorporate into their practice the concept of empathy as advanced by its early theorists and researchers, social scientists continued to explore and experiment with the concept. By 1962 Barrett-Lennard had distinguished between empathic recognition—recognizing the perceptions or feelings of the other person, and empathic inference—"sensing or inferring the implied or indirectly expressed content" of the other person (p. 3). The same theorist (1965) delineated his "Significant Aspects of a Helping Relationship" in 1963, one of which was empathic understanding. "Empathy implies that you appreciate how the other person inwardly feels, how things *are* to him; but it does not mean that his thoughts or feelings or troubles become yours" (p. 2).

Katz, the psychoanalyst, discussed the nature and uses of empathy in a 1963 publication. In it he considered a variety of theories of empathy including those of Lipps, Freud, Mead, and Moreno. Katz asked the question "to what extent is the empathic skill a primitive, biological capacity and to what extent is it a combination of innate and learned behavior?" (p. 55). He concluded from the work of Freud and Mead that it is "a combination of biological endowment and social experience" (p. 77). Over twenty years later researchers studying twins in Canada and Great Britain found that "identical twins are similar to each other in altruism, empathy and nurturance and that fraternal twins tend to be quite different from one another" (Zuckerman, 1985, p. 80).

In the 1960s a considerable number of theorists from a variety of orientations—psychoanalysis, client-centered, eclectic, existential, and behavioristic—were emphasizing the importance of empathy on the part of the therapist (Truax, 1966, p. 8; Carkhuff, 1969b, p. 11). However, in 1965, Eysenck published the results of his second survey of the effectiveness of psychotherapy, and found it small or nonexistent. In 1970 and again in 1977 and 1983, Gladstein maintained that, despite claims for the positive effect of empathy on client outcomes, the evidence in this regard was equivocal (p. 467).

For the purposes of a scale used to measure degrees of empathy, Truax and Carkhuff (1967) defined accurate empathy in general as involving " . . . both the therapist's *sensitivity to current* feelings and his *verbal facility to communicate this understanding* in a language attuned to the client's current feelings" (p. 46). These psychotherapists attempted to bring together emerging behavioral therapy and traditional psychotherapy. Truax and Carkhuff perceived counselors high in empathy, warmth, and genuineness as more effective in psychotherapy because they were potential positive reinforcers for clients, who increased client positive self-reinforcement, decreased anxiety, increased client positive affect and positive reinforcement from others (p. 161).

Stotland defined empathy in 1971 as "an observer reacting emotionally because he perceives that another is experiencing or about to experience an emotion" (Stotland et al., 1978, p. 12). This definition allows for any type of emotional response from the observer. In 1978 Stotland et al. defined empathy

> . . . as a human process, an emotional contagion that can occur whenever two or more people meet and communicate . . . a process shaped by all the variables of the social situation including the status, perceived similarity, and previous interaction of the participants, as well as by the personal orientation of the empathizer—this person's expectancies and aroused emotions (p. 27).

In addition to those who concentrated on the emotional nature of empathy, there were others, as has been indicated, who emphasized cognitive empathy—"intellectually taking the role or the perspective of another person" (Gladstein, 1983, p. 468). Still others viewed empathy as encompassing both cognitive and affective aspects.

EMPATHY AND HELPING

Attempts have been made to determine the level of professionals' empathic ability. For example, Khajavi and Hekmat (1971) found that members of a professional psychiatric team rated higher on empathy than surgeons, but there were no significant differences among psychiatrists (who scored lowest), social workers, psychiatric nurses, activity therapists, and psychologists (who rated highest). The same authors determined that residency in psychiatry did not increase empathy. Truax et al. (1974) reported perceived empathy levels for professionals and found registered nurses on a level with manufacturing plant supervisors. Peitchinis (1972) indicated the generally poor performance of nurses in counseling but indicated that these professionals were attempting to improve their interpersonal skills. Kalisch (1971a, 1971b) considered her empathy training program as the first one conducted with nursing personnel. There have been many since then for nursing staff and students. Most of these are fashioned after training programs developed in counseling and psychotherapy. Rogers had presented a very explicit approach to counselor training in 1957 (Truax and Carkhuff, 1967). Carkhuff's (1969a, 1969b) programs have been used by many, but the research offered in support of Carkhuff's (1969a, 1969b) training programs has been criticized severely by Lambert and De Julio (1977).

There has been much theorizing and considerable research on empathy in education, mental health, corrections, health care, and rehabilitation. In the past two decades some researchers have directed their study to the concept of altruistic helping in emergency or stressful situations. In 1924 Allport had argued that sympathetic emotions.aroused by those who suffer, led mainly to the removal of one's own unpleasant state rather than that of the sufferer (Gladstein, 1983, p. 474). Over fifty years later it was being maintained that another's distress may cause emotional contagion or empathic distress with a tendency to act; whether one does or not depends on circumstances (Ibid.). In 1970, Aderman and Berkowitz considered it desirable to pursue Aronfreed's contention that "altruism is generally motivated by empathy" (p. 147). Liebhart (1972) referred to the assumption that observing an individual in distress causes emotional arousal "which is more intense the more the observer empathizes with the victim" (p. 404). It may be that a number of situational and personality variables determine whether one will attempt to rescue a victim. Assistance is assumed by some to be motivated to rid oneself of an empathy-produced unpleasant emotional state. Krebs (1975) determined that individuals with "the strongest empathic reactions toward another were most willing to help him, even though it meant jeopardizing their own behavior" (p. 1144). However Krebs' work did not demonstrate that "all altruistic behavior is mediated by empathic reactions; nor . . . that all behavior that is mediated by empathy is altruistic" (p. 1145).

An alternative view of empathy—a cognitive one, viewing the world as the other sees it—also has been associated with motivation for helping. It has been suggested (Feshbach, 1975) that rather than being either an emotional or cognitive factor the two types of empathy may interact. A Kansas group (Coke et al., 1978) has proposed a two–stage model of empathic mediation of helping:

(a) Taking the perspective of a person in need tends to increase one's empathic emotional response;
(b) empathic emotion in turn increases motivation to see that person's need reduced (p. 753).

The theorists point to considerable research for the first premise, but much less so for the second. They add a third for which they know of no empirical evidence "that perspective taking affects helping only as a result of its effect on one's empathic emotional response." Coke et al. (1978) view their research as supporting their two-stage model of empathic helping but not as conclusive evidence. Nevertheless they think it would be a mistake to assume people help each other for egoistic desires to reduce their own distress, for in their view, "empathic emotion may produce an altruistic desire to have the stress of others reduced" (p. 765).

Three years later, a Texas group, Archer et al. (1981) proposed that the model of Coke et al. (1978) encompasses other factors— an individual's tendency to empathize, a stable dispositional factor, and a situational factor, which is the potential for receiving evaluation from others or the potential for social evaluation. Both of these factors should increase helping according to Archer et al. About the same time the Kansas group (Batson et al., 1981) discussed helping as an altruistically or egoistically motivated act and continued to experiment with their empathy–altruism hypothesis. The latter led to the suggestion that "empathic motivation for helping may be truly altruistic" (p. 302). Further evidence of support was reported in 1982 (Toi and Batson). In 1983 Batson et al. disagreed with the suggestion made by the group from Texas (Archer et al., 1981) for augmenting their empathy–altruism hypothesis. Such were considered unnecessary.

Davis (1983) viewed his work as demonstrating that "individual differences in empathy can influence empathic emotion and personal distress, above and beyond the influence of situational factors" (p. 167). These differences were found to be in emotional empathy, not cognitive empathy, and so support what Davis calls the "multidimensional nature of empathy"—its cognitive and emotional aspects. Most of the research on empathy and altruistic helping has been conducted in the laboratory; it will be interesting to see if the conclusions are upheld in actual emergency situations. In 1984, Archer attempted to promote a reconciliation with Batson and his colleagues suggesting that their two approaches to empathy and helping could be complementary and that both could be correct in part.

Another factor in helping is religion, which has been investigated. Watson et al. (1984) envision their work as supporting Batson's (1983) view of empathy as a component of religiosity. More research is needed to determine whether empathic motivation is influenced by religiosity—helping behavior—and whether this motivation is egoistic or altruistic. Batson (1983) has suggested that there may be "an innate kin-specific altruistic impulse in humans. . . ." (p. 1383). The possibility that telepathy plays a role in empathy is not excluded by Szalita (1976). However, she does admit that the effect may be an instantaneous response to nonverbal cues (p. 148).

OTHER DEVELOPMENTS

In 1981, Barrett-Lennard delineated "a sequence of distinct stages involved in empathic interaction" (p. 91). This sequence encompassed a five-step empathy cycle as follows:

1) A actively attends B who hopes A is receptive (Empathic Act)
2) A resonates to B so that the latter's experience becomes known to A (Empathic Resonation)
3) A shows felt awareness of B's experience (Expressed Empathy)
4) B has a sense of A's understanding (Received Empathy)
5) B continues expression providing A with information to confirm perception of B's experience and to confirm B's perception of A as understanding. The cycle then reverts to Step Two (p. 94).

Empathy is seen as a "process sequence in actual interaction contexts" (p. 97). Each step of the process must follow in order. Each phase of the sequence requires different methods of measuring it. Gladstein (1983) thinks that emotional contagion as discussed in developmental and social psychology needs to be added to Barrett-Lennard's empathy cycle. The latter's five-stage empathy sequence is interesting since Kurtz and Grummon (1972) had drawn attention almost a decade earlier to the variety of ways empathy was conceptualized and measured in attempts to determine its effect on client outcomes. They wondered whether one variable or several different variables were involved in the same term—empathy.

From an analysis of the literature on empathy in the fields of developmental and social psychology, Gladstein (1983) determined that these subdisciplines differ not only between themselves but also with counseling/psychotherapy on empathy definitions and measures. However, all identify both emotional and cognitive or role-taking types of empathy. As a consequence of his study, Gladstein (1983) proposes that:

> First, empathy should be viewed as a multistage interpersonal process that can involve emotional contagion, identification, and role taking. Second, empathy in children is probably different from empathy in adolescence and adulthood. Third, empathy can but does not necessarily lead to helping behavior. Last, empathy in counseling/psychotherapy can be helpful in certain stages, with certain clients, and for certain goals. However, at other times it can interfere with positive outcomes (p. 467).

In a fairly recent 90-page exposition on the relationship in counseling and psychotherapy, Gelso and Carter (1985) made only very brief reference to empathy. Their views of the counseling relationship are based on psychoanalysis, humanism, learning approaches, and conditioning theory.

A century has passed since Lipps described and labelled Einfühlung—Titchener's empathy. It is now thirty years since Rogers (1957) proposed that empathy was a crucial ingredient in counseling and psychotherapy. Gladstein viewed the evidence bearing on this notion in 1983 and concluded "it is not clear what part empathy actually has in producing positive outcomes" (p. 480). But he added that much has been learned about empathy's various aspects and stages. In nursing, La Monica (1979) has pointed to the needs to obtain a valid empathy measuring instrument and to investigate whether nurses being empathic makes a difference to what she calls nursing care outcomes, or what one would think of as patient outcomes. These prescriptions seem applicable today.

REFERENCES

Aderman, D., & Berkowitz, L. (1970). Observational set, empathy, and helping. *Journal of Personality and Social Psychology, 14*(2), 141–148.

Allport, G. W. (1937). *Personality: A psychological interpretation.* New York: Henry Holt.

Archer, R. L., Diaz-Loving, R., Gollwitzer, P. M., Davis, M. H. and Foushee, H. C. (1981). The role of dispositional empathy and social evaluation in the empathic mediation of helping. *Journal of Personality and Social Psychology, 40*(4), 787–796.

Archer, R. L. (1984). The farmer and the cowman should be friends: An attempt at reconciliation with Batson, Coke, and Pych. *Journal of Personality and Social Psychology, 46*(3), 709–711.

Barrett-Lennard, G. T. (1962). Dimensions of therapist response as causal factors in therapeutic change. *Psychological Monographs, 76*(43) (whole number 562).

Barrett-Lennard, G. T. (July–August, 1965). Significant aspects of a helping relationship. *Canada's Mental Health, 13*, (Supplement No. 47).

Barrett-Lennard, G. T. (1981). The empathy cycle: Refinement of a nuclear concept. *Journal of Counseling Psychology, 28*(2), 91–100.

Bates, B. (1974). Doctor and nurse: Changing roles and relations. *Nursing Digest II,* (8), 70–75.

Batson, C. D., Duncan, B. D., Ackerman, P., Buckley, T., and Birch, K. (1981). Is empathic emotion a source of altruistic motivation? *Journal of Personality and Social Psychology, 40*(2), 290–302.

Batson, C. D. (1983). Sociobiology and the role of religion in promoting prosocial behavior: An alternative view. *Journal of Personality and Social Psychology, 45*(6), 1380–1385.

Batson, C. D., Coke, J. S., Pych, V. (1983). Limits on the two-stage model of empathic mediation of helping: A reply to Archer, Diaz-Loving, Gollwitzer, Davis and Foushee. *Journal of Personality and Social Psychology, 45*(4), 895–898.

Bettelheim, B. (1962). To nurse and to nurture. *Nursing Forum 1,* 61–76.

Bird, B. (1955). *Talking with patients.* Philadelphia: J. B. Lippincott.

Bird, B. (1973). *Talking with patients.* (2nd ed.). Toronto: J. B. Lippincott.

Calnan, J. (1983). *Talking with patients: A guide to good practice.* London: William Heinemann.

Carkhuff, R. R. (1969a). *Helping and human relations: A primer for lay and professional helpers: Vol. 1, Selection and training.* New York: Holt, Rinehart and Winston.

Carkhuff, R. R. (1969b). *Helping and human relations: A primer for lay and professional helpers: Vol. 2, Practice and research.* New York: Holt, Rinehart and Winston.

Cassell, E. J. (1985). *Talking with patients: Vol. I. The theory of doctor–patient communication.* Cambridge, MA: MIT Press.

Coke, J. S., Batson, C. D., McDavis, K. (1978). Empathic mediation of helping: A two-stage model. *Journal of Personality and Social Psychology*, 36(7), 752–766.

Davis, M. H. (1983). The effects of dispositional empathy on emotional reactions and helping: A multidimensional approach. *Journal of Personality*, 51(2), 167–184.

Dymond, R. F. (1949). A scale for measurement of empathic ability. *Journal of Consulting Psychology*, 13, 127–133.

Dymond, R. F. (1950). Personality and empathy. *Journal of Consulting Psychology*, 14, 343–350.

Elizur, A., & Rosenheim E. (1982). Empathy and attitudes among medical students: The effects of group experience. *Journal of Medical Education*, 57(9), 675–683.

Engel, G. L., & Morgan, W. L., Jr. (1973). *Interviewing the patient*. Philadelphia: W. B. Saunders.

Evang, K. (1960). *Health service, society and medicine*. London: Oxford University Press.

Eysenck, H. J. (1952). The effects of psychotherapy: An evaluation. *Journal of Consulting Psychology*, 16, 319–324.

Eysenck, H. J. (1965). The effects of psychotherapy. *International Journal of Psychiatry*, 1(1), 99–142.

Feshbach, N. D. (1975). Empathy in children: Some theoretical and empirical considerations. *The Counseling Psychologist*, 5(2), 25–30.

Fischer, J. (1976). *The effectiveness of social casework*. Springfield, IL: Charles C. Thomas.

Freud, S. (1959). *Group psychology and the analysis of the ego* (rev. ed.). New York: Liveright. 2nd Impression 1967 (Translated and Edited by J. Strachey) Originally published 1921.

Gelso, C. J. and Carter, J. A. (1985). The Relationship in counseling and psychotherapy. *The Counseling Psychologist*, 13(2), 155–244.

Gladstein, G. A. (1970). Is empathy important in counseling? *Personnel and Guidance Journal*, 48, 823–827.

Gladstein, G. A. (1977). Empathy and Counseling Outcome: An Empirical and Conceptual Review. *Counseling Psychologist*, 6(4), 70–79.

Gladstein, G. A. (1983). Understanding empathy: Integrating counseling, developmental, and social psychology perspectives. *Journal of Counseling Psychology*, 30(4), 467–482.

Greenson, R. R. (1967). *The technique and practice of psychoanalysis* (Vol. 1). New York: International Universities Press.

Hackney, H. (1978). The evolution of empathy. *Personnel and Guidance Journal*, 57, 35–39.

Henderson, V. (1964). The nature of nursing. *American Journal of Nursing*, 64(8), 62–68.

Holmes, M. J., & Werner, J. A. (1966). *Psychiatric nursing in a therapeutic community*. New York: Macmillan.

Jourard, S. M. (1961). Roles that sicken and transactions that heal. *Canadian Nurse, 57*(7), 628–634.

Kalisch, B. J. (1971a). An experiment in the development of empathy in nursing students. *Nursing Research, 20*(3), 202–211.

Kalisch, B. J. (1971b). Strategies for developing nurse empathy. *Nursing Outlook, 19*(11), 714–718.

Katz, R. L. (1963). *Empathy, its nature and uses.* Glencoe: Free Press.

Khajavi, F., Hekmat, H. (1971). A comparative study of empathy. *Archives General Psychiatry, 25,* 490–493.

Kozier, B. B., & Du Gas, B. W. (1967). *Fundamentals of patient care: A comprehensive approach to nursing.* Philadelphia: Saunders.

Krebs, D. (1975). Empathy and altruism. *Journal of Personality and Social Psychology, 32*(6), 1134–1146.

Kurtz, R. R., & Grummon, D. L. (1972). Different approaches to the measurement of therapist empathy and their relationship to therapy's outcomes. *Journal of Consulting and Clinical Psychology, 39*(1), 106–115.

Lambert, M. J. and De Julio, S. S. (1977). Outcome research in Carkhuff's human resource development training programs: Where is the donut? *The Counseling Psychologist, 6*(4), 79–86.

La Monica, E. L. (1979). Empathy in nursing practice. *Issues in Mental Health Nursing, 2,* 1–13.

Liebhart, E. H. (1972). Empathy and emergency helping: The effects of personality, self-concern, and acquaintance. *Journal of Experimental Social Psychology, 8,* 404–411.

Lockerby, F. K. (1968). *Communication for nurses.* St. Louis, MO: C. V. Mosby.

Nordmark, M. T., & Rohweder A. W. (1959). *Science principles applied to nursing: A reference for nurse educators.* Philadelphia: J. B. Lippincott.

Orlando, I. J. (1961). *The dynamic nurse–patient relationship: Function, process and principles.* New York: Putnam.

Peitchinis, J. (1972). Therapeutic effectiveness of counseling by nursing personnel. *Nursing Research, 21*(2), 138–148.

Peitchinis, J. A. (1976). *Staff–Patient Communication in the Health Services.* New York: Springer Publishing Co.

Penfield, W. (March, 1966). [Letter to the editor] *Dalhousie Medical Journal, 19*(3), 87.

Peplau, H. E., (1952). *Interpersonal relations in nursing.* New York: Putnam.

Perlman, H. H. (Ed.) (1969). *Helping: Charlotte Towle on social work and social casework.* Chicago: University of Chicago Press.

Rogers, C. R. (1942). *Counseling and psychotherapy: Newer concepts in practice.* Cambridge, MA: Riverside Press.

Rogers, C. R. (1951). *Client-centered therapy: Its current practice, implications and theory.* Chicago: Houghton Mifflin.

Rogers, C. R. (1956). A counseling approach to human problems. *American Journal of Nursing, 56*(8), 994–997.

Rogers, C. R. (1957). The necessary and sufficient conditions of therapeutic personality change. *Journal of Consulting Psychology, 21,* 95–103.

Rogers, C. R. (March, 1962). Characteristics of a helping relationship. *Canada's Mental Health, 10* (Supplement No. 27). (Published in 1958 in Personnel and Guidance Journal.)

Rogers, C. R., & Dymond R. F. (1954). *Psychotherapy and personality change: Coordinated research studies in the client-centered approach.* Chicago: The University of Chicago Press.

Ruesch, J. (1961). *Therapeutic communication.* New York: Norton.

Speroff, B. J. (1956). Empathy is important in nursing. *Nursing Outlook, 4*(6), 326–328.

Stewart, D. (1956). *Preface to empathy.* New York: Philosophical Library.

Stotland, E., Mathews Jr., K. E., Sherman, S. E., Hansson, R., & Richardson, B. Z. (1978). *Empathy, fantasy and helping.* Beverly Hills, CA: Sage.

Streit-Forest, U. (1982). Differences in empathy: A preliminary analysis. *Journal of Medical Education, 57*(1), 65–67.

Szalita, A. B. (1976). Some thoughts on empathy. *Psychiatry, 39,* 142–152.

Szasz, T. S., & Hollender, M. (1956). A contribution to the philosophy of medicine: The basic models of the doctor–patient relationship. *Archives of Internal Medicine, 97,* 585–592.

Taylor, C. (1970). *In horizontal orbit: Hospitals and the cult of efficiency.* New York: Holt, Rinehart & Winston.

Toi, M. and Batson, C. D. (1982). More evidence that empathy is a souce of altruistic motivation. *Journal of Personality and Social Psychology, 43*(2), 281–292.

Truax, C. B. (1966). *Counseling and psychotherapy: Process and outcome.* University of Arkansas: Arkansas Rehabilitation Research and Training Center.

Truax, C. B., & Carkhuff, R. R. (1967). *Toward effective counseling and psychotherapy: Training and practice.* Chicago: Aldine.

Truax, C. B., Altmann, H., & Millis, Jr., W. A. (1974). Therapeutic relationships provided by various professionals. *Journal of Community Psychology, 2*(1), 33–36.

Watson, P. J., Hood, R. W., Morris, R. J., & Hall, J. R. (1984). Empathy, religious orientation, and social desirability. *The Journal of Psychology, 117,* 211–216.

Wiedenbach, E. (1964). *Clinical nursing: A helping art.* New York: Springer Publishing Co.

Witthower, E. D., & Warnes, H. (Eds.) (1977). *Psychosomatic medicine: Its clinical applications.* New York: Harper & Row.

Zuckerman, D. (1985). Can genes help helping? *Psychology Today, 19*(3), 80.

Part II

Empathy: A Personality Factor and a Skill

The debate as to whether empathy is a personality disposition or a skill continues today as it has in the past. Johnson, in Chapter 4, examines empathy as it is derived from the personality, and in Chapter 5 Gazda and Evans present the view that empathy is both an attitude and a learned skill. A theoretical model of empathy based on both orientations is put forward in Chapter 6 This model has influenced the examination of empathy which is described later in Part Three of the book.

The measurement of empathy has been a thorny problem for both practitioners and researchers. Chapter 7 discusses the major means of measurement found in a review of the published literature, with an analysis of the advantages and difficulties associated with each type.

4

Empathy as a Personality Disposition

John A. Johnson

MacKay's initial chapter of this book demonstrates the complexity of the empathy construct by reviewing various definitions and conceptualizations of empathy. The present chapter analyzes empathy as a personality disposition. Empathy—like any personality disposition—possesses four levels of meaning. These four levels of meaning are: (1) global, evaluative impressions about an actor perceived by an audience; (2) regularities in an actor's behavior that are responsible for these global impressions; (3) conscious desires and plans that guide an actor's behavior; and (4) latent structures responsible for an actor's desires and plans. These four layers of personality help explain, respectively, (1) how empathy affects the helping relationship; (2) which specific behaviors can be taught in empathy training programs; (3) why people act empathically or unempathically in social interaction; and (4) the natural constraints on empathy development in training programs.

CLASSICAL DEFINITIONS OF PERSONALITY

Understanding empathy as a personality disposition requires an understanding of the general nature of personality. Therefore, the first half of this chapter is devoted to clarifying the general nature of personality. This excursus may seem to take us somewhat far afield of the topic of empathy, but is absolutely necessary for understanding the nature of empathy as a personality disposition.

Just as empathy possesses numerous definitions, so does personality. In fact, Allport (1937, Chapter 2) identified 50 different definitions of personality. Fortunately, Allport reduced the 50 definitions to two central meanings of personality—that of outer appearance and that of inner (essential) nature. Most personality and social psychologists continue to use one or both of these two central definitions (Baumeister, 1986; Hogan, 1976; MacKinnon, 1944).

Viewing personality as outer appearance derives directly from the Latin term *persona,* a theatrical mask worn to signify an actor's role in a play. Defining personality in this manner has several ramifications. First, this definition creates the dramaturgical metaphor for social interaction (Goffman, 1959), that is, it suggests that we are all actors performing to create certain impressions on our audiences. Second, it suggests that we can "change personalities" for different audiences, much as Greek actors changed masks for different roles. Third, it raises questions concerning sincerity and genuineness, because "putting on an act" is generally taken to mean pretending to be someone other than who one really is. Finally, the mask notion of personality implies the existence of a "hidden" person behind the mask.

Viewing personality as a hidden assemblage of inner personal qualities has been the mainstay of Freud and the depth psychologists. This perspective suggests alternative implications to those suggested by the mask definition. First, it suggests that we possess intrinsic personality traits that exist apart from our transactions with other people. Second, it implies the stability and relative immutability of personality (i.e., the masks may change, but the actor does not). Third, the existence of a stable self implies that sincerity is possible. Finally, it provides a specific definition of sincerity: people are sincere to the degree that their outer actions accurately reflect their inner psychological traits.

THE SOCIAL PSYCHOLOGICAL CONCEPTUALIZATION OF PERSONALITY

Experimental social psychology has developed its own perspective on the relationship between personality-as-outer-appearances (dramaturgical view) and personality-as-inner-psychic-qualities (depth psychology view). Experimental social psychology— essentially a form of stimulus-response behaviorism (Hendrick, 1977)—has sought to identify specific, concrete, observable actor behaviors that serve as stimuli affecting the perceptual responses of the audience. Thus we get from experimental social psychology a fine-grained analysis of actor characteristics that influence personality-qua-appearance.

The experimental approach has successfully revealed how specific actor characteristics (facial features, eye contact, speech mannerisms, body posture, etc.) influence an audience's perception of the actor's friendliness, likeability, dominance, trustworthiness, and so forth (Buck, Miller, & Caul, 1974; Ekman, 1965; Exline & Fehr, 1978; Kleinke, 1975; Kraut & Johnston, 1979; Secord, 1958). For example, people appear to be friendly when they exhibit "friendly behaviors"—smiling, making appropriate eye contact, and so forth.

The consensus of the research cited above is that an audience forms its initial impressions of an actor's personality by rapidly synthesizing bits of verbal and nonverbal information into an overall personality portrait. Like all perceptual reactions, the process of forming first impressions is automatic; that is to say, the synthesis of sensory stimuli into an overall personality impression is nonvoluntary and occurs below the observer's level of awareness. The actor's sincerity or honesty is determined in part by comparing verbal and nonverbal messages, particularly *involuntary* nonverbal messages (Ekman & Friesen, 1974; Kraut, 1978). Much of impression formation therefore can be said to be governed by principles beyond the rational, voluntary control of either actor or observer.

The first contribution, then, of experimental social psychology, has been to explain how immediate outer appearances are generated automatically by specific behaviors. A second contribution of social psychology is an explication of how an audience infers stable, *inner* personality dispositions from continued observations of behavioral acts. This area, known as *attribution theory*, suggests that judgments of inner personality dispositions are rarely arrived at in a calculated manner (Heider, 1958). More often, people infer general personality traits unconsciously according to certain tacit rules.

A third and final contribution offered by experimental social psychology has been to demonstrate individual differences in the ability to form accurate personality impressions from behavioral observations. Among the characteristics of "good judges" of personality is, interestingly, empathy (Mills & Hogan, 1973; Borman, 1979). More will be said about empathy and accuracy in person perception later.

In summary, the social–psychological perspective on the relationship between inner personality and outer appearances gives us three valuable insights. First, first impressions of personality are formed rapidly, automatically, and below the level of awareness of both actor and audience. Second, inferences about inner personality from behavioral data are also made spontaneously and unconsciously. Third, some people judge personality from behavioral observations more accurately than others, and one of the characteristics of a good judge is empathy.

FROM TRAIT DESCRIPTIONS TO STRUCTURAL EXPLANATIONS

Social psychologists have successfully explained why people consistently create specific impressions on each other. Apparently, each of us is consistent in his/her mannerisms (particularly nonverbal mannerisms), and these mannerisms are automatically perceived in specific ways, leading to consistent personality impressions.

What behavioristically oriented social psychologists cannot explain, however, are our consistent behavioral mannerisms. If external stimuli totally controlled our behavior, then our external environment would have to remain perfectly constant to produce consistent behavior. The fact that people exhibit consistent behavioral mannerisms across different environmental contexts repudiates the behavioristic, social–psychological view.

Where, then, are we to look for an explanation of the consistent behavioral mannerisms that lead to consistent personality impressions? Alston (1975) suggests looking to the *inner structure* of the actor. More specifically, he claims that regularities in behavior (which he calls *trait dispositions* or "T-concepts") can be explained with *purposive-cognitive* ("PC")-concepts. PC-concepts include three basic types of inner psychological determinants: *desires* (feelings of longing for particular goals), *beliefs* (cognitive schemata outlining the most promising ways to achieve desired goals), and *abilities* (the capacity to perform behaviors required in the desire–belief plan). Thus, Mary may behave empathically because she desires cooperation from others, believes that empathic behavior is the best way to obtain cooperation, and has the ability to behave empathically.

Alston admits that his explanation of intentional behavior in terms of desires, beliefs, and abilities is quite common-sensical ("in its gross outlines is familiar to all of us since childhood" are his exact words—1975, p. 24). A more complete, "scientific" view of inner personality requires an explanation of the relationship between conscious desires and plans and the deep causal structures that ultimately guide conscious activity. One conceptualization of this deep structure is the *talent* construct (cf. Newman & Newman, 1980).

Talents can be regarded as the neurophysiological potential or capacity for executing specific behavior patterns. The presence of a talent for a specific behavior means that, given the opportunity, the talented person will (a) learn the behavior quickly and effortlessly, (b) eventually execute the behavior gracefully and skillfully at high levels of performance, and (c) receive intrinsic pleasure from engaging in the behavior. Drawing an analogy between "personality talent" and athletic talent will further clarify how personality develops.

Let us use the development of basketball talent as an example. Some basketball players learn skills quickly and effortlessly and develop these skills to a high level. Others struggle when learning and never perform very well. What coaches call a "born" basketball player apparently possesses a certain amount of innate (genetically determined) talent that facilitates learning and allows for high levels of performance.

Basketball skills, although influenced by genes, do not appear full-blown in children; they develop through practice—repeated practice. Coaches drill players until the basic moves in the sport become unconscious habits. Skilled athletes (or musicians) will tell you that consciously thinking about their motor movements disrupts the grace and accuracy of their performances. Initially, players must think about every newly learned set of movements, but eventually these conscious plans become unconscious cognitive programs. When a basketball player tells himself "turn-around jump shot," an automatic sequence of movements occurs (cf. Lennenberg's, 1967, concept of language automatisms).

Personality talents—including empathy—are very similar to basketball skills in this regard. Naturally empathic persons gravitate toward fields such as counseling because they learn counseling skills easily and enjoy counseling activities. After counselors have become skilled through hundreds of hours of practice, they can tell themselves "do Rogerian counseling," and a smooth pattern of reflective listening and empathic responding is executed. If the counselor for some reason were to suddenly become self-conscious, the flow is disrupted and the performance becomes unnatural, unconvincing, and ungenuine. Likewise, an untrained therapist who lacks a knack (talent) for counseling will probably be seen as less caring than a trained, skilled counselor.

Understanding talents as the origin of "natural" behavior sheds new light on the perception of "authenticity" or "sincerity." When we are "being ourselves" we are executing talent-based, well-practiced behavior patterns. Such performances are fluid and smooth, and are therefore automatically assumed to be authentic (i.e., in correspondence with inner personality) by audiences. In nonrehearsed, unpracticed performances we appear awkward, unnatural, uncoordinated, and ungenuine. Our verbal and nonverbal messages don't jibe, and our real dispositions may leak through (Lippa, 1978).

In addition to quick, effortless learning and high levels of performance, athletic skills and personality talents have in common a pleasant affect that accompanies the performance of the behavior. Athletes play not just to win, but for the sheer kinesthetic pleasure of the sport. A genuine basketball player will feel an urge to dribble and shoot the ball all year, not just during the season. Likewise, people feel an urgency to seek out opportunities to execute the behaviors that satisfy their cardinal inner personality dispositions—their personality talents. Conscious desires are activated (in part) by these deeper underlying talents.

The notion of personality talents therefore explains ultimately *why* people exhibit consistent behavior patterns (which, in turn, lead to consistent personality impressions). Predisposing, innate structures in the nervous system (talents) make certain activities intrinsically easy to execute, and the pleasure derived from executing the activities reinforces the person to repeat and practice the activity until it becomes an unconscious habit.

Although personality talents possess both motor skill and cognitive qualities, they are identical to neither athletic skills nor purely intellectual skills. Personality talents always develop within a social context and are intimately linked to outer personality impressions. Personality talents are essentially raw materials without form. Young children learn to shape these raw materials into the form of *roles* by imitating admired role models. Empathy—the ability to take the perspective of another person—is a crucial part of learning to play roles. For successful role learning, the young actor must be able to evaluate, from the perspective of the audience, the impression he or she is making upon that audience.

SUMMARY OF THE GENERAL NATURE OF PERSONALITY

In summary, personality dispositions can be analyzed into four tiers according to the perspective of the observer. The general public or audience reacts to their *impressions* of actors. Social psychologists have identified *specific behaviors* that create these impressions. The actors themselves explain their behaviors in terms of *desires, beliefs,* and *abilities* (e.g., "I paint because I enjoy it, I think it's the best way to express myself, and I'm good at it.") Finally, the personality theorists make hypotheses about predisposing genetic and neuronal *structures* that facilitate the social learning experiences that lead to the actors' desires, beliefs, and abilities.

This perspective therefore explains audience impressions in terms of behaviors, behaviors in terms of actors' desires, beliefs, and abilities, and these actors' qualities in terms of underlying physiology and developmental patterns. This perspective also stresses the interaction of outer and inner factors in personality development. The roles that actors learn to play are formed jointly by predisposing talents and the influence of role models. Finally, an actor's success at role-playing is a function of unself-conscious authenticity, which audiences evaluate constantly by the act's degree of effortlessness and coherence of verbal and nonverbal components. These general principles will now be applied to an analysis of *empathy*.

IMPRESSIONS OF EMPATHIC PERSONS

Do empathic persons create similar impressions on different audiences? Hogan (1969) addressed this question by selecting 50 items whose content was directly relevant to empathy from the 100-item California Q-set, an instrument designed to provide a comprehensive description of personality impressions (Block, 1961). Hogan then asked a group of nonpsychologists and a group of psychology graduate students to sort the Q-set items to describe a "highly empathic man," using the following dictionary definition of empathy, "the intellectual or imaginative apprehension of another's condition or state of mind without actually experiencing that person's feelings." The estimated reliabilities of the composite Q-sorts in the groups were .94 and .90, and the corrected correlation between group Q-sort composites was .93. This indicates a high level of agreement within groups and between lay and psychological audiences on the impressions generated by an empathic person.

Encouraged by these results, Hogan (1969) requested a group of professional psychologists and advanced graduate students at the University of California at Berkeley to describe a highly empathic man with the full 100-item Q-set. Again, a highly reliable (.94) composite was found. The five items from the composite Q-sort selected by the group as *most characteristic* of an empathic man were as follows:

1. Is skilled in social techniques of imaginative play, pretending, and humor.
2. Seems to be aware of the impression he makes on others.
3. Evaluates the motivation of others in interpreting situations.
4. Has insight into own motives and behavior.
5. Is socially perceptive of a wide range of interpersonal cues.

In summary, empathic people impress us, first of all, as *perceptive* or *insightful*. The eight items from the composite Q-sort selected as *quite characteristic* of an empathic man were as follows (Hogan, 1967):

1. Appears to have a high degree of intellectual capacity.
2. Is introspective and concerned with self as an object.
3. Behaves in a sympathetic manner.
4. Is turned to for advice and reassurance.
5. Has warmth; has the capacity for close relationships, compassionate.
6. Responds to humor.
7. Able to see to the heart of important problems.
8. Emphasizes communication through action and non-verbal behavior.

Several of these items (1, 2, 7) again reflect perceptiveness and insightfulness, but a new theme is found in items 3, 4, 5, and 6. These items indicate that empathic people impress us as *sympathetic, helpful, warm, compassionate*, and *good-natured*.

Hogan's results were replicated by La Monica (1980), who solicited descriptions of a highly empathic person from female psychology graduate students, nurses, and university professors. Both the *perceptiveness* and *compassion* themes can be seen in the five descriptions showing the highest loadings in a factor analysis of descriptions she gathered:

1. Seems to understand another person's state of being.
2. Helps a person work through his situation and his problems/concerns.
3. Understands the "human" situation.
4. Shows consideration for a person's feelings and reactions.
5. Understands the problems of others by putting herself in their place.

The personality impressions listed above were generated by professionals in the fields of psychology and nursing. Hogan (1969) also provides data on the impressions of nonpsychologists of the empathic person. From the personality archives at Berkeley, Hogan selected 64 self-report inventory items that tended to be endorsed by subjects whose Q-sort profiles resembled the Q-sort of the "highly empathic man." This 64-item, true/false Empathy Scale was administered to 103 fraternity men, who also rated each other on the 300-word Adjective Check List (ACL) (Gough & Heilbrun, 1965). The ten words most descriptive of high scorers on the Empathy Scale were: pleasant, charming, friendly, dreamy, cheerful, sociable, sentimental, imaginative, discreet, and tactful. The ten words most descriptive of low scorers were: cruel, cold, quarrelsome, hostile, bitter, unemotional, unkind, hard-hearted, argumentative, and opinionated. These ACL ratings seem to confirm both the perceptive and compassionate aspects of empathy, although the compassionate aspect is better represented.

That empathic persons impress others as perceptive and compassionate explains how empathy generates trust, confidence, and openness in the patient–caretaker relationship. A patient who sees his caretaker as perceptive and compassionate is likely to say, "This person understands me and is sensitive to my condition. She can help me because she can really tell what's going on with me and care enough for me to make me feel better. I can be frank with this person, and I trust her judgment enough to go along with what she says."

Caretaker perceptiveness therefore generates in the patient confidence in the caretaker's ability to do the right thing, which increases the likelihood of patient compliance. Caretaker compassion reduces apprehension in the patient, which generates a willingness in the patient to reveal openly sensitive material. Note, however, that neither perceptiveness nor compassion alone is sufficient to facilitate compliance and communication; both are essential. A caretaker who is perceptive but cold will seem invasive and cause the patient to clam up. A caretaker who is compassionate but imperceptive will appear inept and unworthy of compliance. Furthermore, verbal and nonverbal caretaker messages must be congruent to generate positive impressions in the helping relationship (Graves & Robinson, 1976).

BEHAVIORAL REGULARITIES
OF EMPATHIC PERSONS

Counselors have been cataloging for many years the specific behaviors underlying empathic impressions in order to teach these behaviors to persons desiring to appear empathic in the helping relationship. Buchheimer and Balogh (1961) have categorized types of verbal leads in terms of their effect on the person being counseled. Compassion, acceptance, and support are communicated by (1) silence or statements indicating patience and receptiveness (e.g., "Take your time, there's no rush"); (2) statements of reassurance (e.g., "That's, okay, I'm with you, you're not alone in this"); or (3) restatements of manifest content or feeling (e.g., "You are saying . . . " or "You say you feel . . . "). Accurate understanding is communicated by reflection—a paraphrasing of content or feeling (e.g., "In other words, you feel . . . ").

Nonverbal behaviors communicating empathy have also been studied and catalogued. D'Augelli (1974) found that the frequency of helpers' head nods influenced impressions of both the helper's warmth and understanding. Tepper and Haase (1978) found that tone of voice and facial expression explained more variance in impressions of empathy than the verbal message, but qualified this conclusion by suggesting that effective messages require a proper balance between verbal and nonverbal messages. Smith-Hanen (1977) found that both arm and leg posture affected impressions of empathy, a significant finding, given that body posture tends to be subject to less voluntary control than facial expression (Ekman & Friesen, 1974).

These catalogs of verbal and nonverbal behaviors that reflect empathy can provide useful basic material for programs designed to teach empathic behavior (cf. Hughes, Carver, & Mackay, Chapter 8 of this volume). Two absolutely essential elements for making empathy training programs work are (a) role-playing practice sessions that simulate actual therapeutic encounters; and (b) opportunities to review videotapes of the role-playing sessions. The practice is necessary to make the empathic responses more fluid, natural, and spontaneous. The videotapes are necessary to help the trainees observe their nonverbal behavior and make it congruent with their verbal behavior. (Recall that "naturalness" and verbal/nonverbal congruence are the two means by which an audience judges the sincerity of the actor; mechanical, incongruent empathic behavior will not be as effective as natural, congruent empathic behavior.)

It is important to keep in mind that videotaping may temporarily disrupt the fluidness and naturalness of trainee behavior by heightening their self-consciousness. That is why continued practice is so essential for developing behavior that appears convincingly empathic. The trainee must practice empathic behavior until it is no longer necessary to monitor his or her responding. Empathy will then become an automatic response and appear to be genuine to the audience.

MOTIVATIONS AND DESIRES
OF EMPATHIC PERSONS

Commitment to any pattern of behavior requires a certain amount of emotional involvement. If behavior is executed merely as a means to an end, it will be neither practiced often nor performed with enthusiasm. Consequently, the behavioral performance will be lackluster and unconvincing. In the case of empathic behavior, the person must genuinely *want* to behave empathically in order to give sincere-sounding, genuine-appearing empathic responses.

A factor analysis of Hogan's Empathy Scale (Johnson, Cheek, & Smither, 1983) sheds some light on the motives underlying empathic behavior. Johnson et al. found four factors in Hogan's scale, which they named *Social Self-Confidence, Even Temperedness, Sensitivity*, and *Nonconformity*. Social Self-Confidence describes an intrinsic interest in interacting with other people. Empathic persons enjoy simply being with others. Even temperedness is best understood as the *absence* of a motive to attract attention to one's self by complaining about one's problems. Even temperedness is a particularly valuable asset for helpers in the medical and health care professions, given that the people they treat *are* normally self-absorbed in their problems.

Johnson et al. consider Sensitivity and Nonconformity to be the two most important facets of Hogan's Empathy Scale. Sensitivity describes an interest in feeling-tones (i.e., aesthetic reactivity) and a concern with social approval. Empathic persons are sensitive to the feelings of others; they feel bad when others hurt. Thus, the Sensitivity factor of empathy is similar to what we normally call *sympathy*—the tendency to feel what others feel. Note, however, that pure sympathy is self-defeating in the therapeutic helping relationship because merely experiencing a patient's negative feelings can immobilize a helper. Sensitivity must be balanced by Even Temperedness. Truly empathic people do not become overwhelmed at the pain of others. Rather, they objectively understand others' feelings in order to help relieve their suffering. Empathic persons find helping others intrinsically satisfying, and they also enjoy receiving gratitude from those they help.

"Nonconformity" is an incompletely accurate label for a rather complex syndrome that includes an interest in novelty and change, liberal political attitudes, and an intraceptive cognitive style (a tendency to think in terms of complex and differentiated interpersonal concepts rather than bias-ridden stereotypes). The motivational aspect of Nonconformity is the interest in novelty and openness to new information. Empathic persons resist jumping to quick conclusions about people, which increases the accuracy of their perceptions of others. Johnson et al. (1983) and Johnson and Worley (1987) suggest that the Nonconformity factor is specifically responsible for accuracy in person perception.

In summary, empathic persons (1) enjoy interacting with others,

(2) are not interested in getting attention by dramatizing their own problems, (3) enjoy receiving gratitude from others for being interested in their feelings, and (4) enjoy getting to know others well. This complex of motivations generally steers the empathic person into one of the helping professions, which Holland (1985) calls *Social* occupations: The cardinal motif of the Social type's life is involvement in others' lives in a positive way (helping, teaching, healing, parenting, serving) because of the intrinsic pleasure of helping others and the rewards of others' appreciation.

Medical personnel sometimes find themselves in a motivational double-bind (cf. Kupfer, Drew, Curtis, & Rubinstein, 1978). Holland (1985) describes these medical occupations as a combination of *Social* and *Investigative* tendencies. That is, medical personnel can be motivated primarily by the Social desire to help others, or by the predominant desire of the Investigative type, which is to solve problems via the scientific method. Investigative types are generally concerned more with ideas than with people; thus we have some medical personnel who do well at diagnosis and labwork, but interact poorly with patients. This implies that empathy training will be most successful for health care personnel whose primary motive is Social, rather than Investigative (cf. Hughes, Carver, & Mackay, Chapter 8, this volume).

DEEP PERSONALITY STRUCTURE
OF EMPATHIC PERSONS

The deepest level of empathy as a personality variable concerns the unobservable structures that enable a person to perform skillfully in an empathic manner. Gazda and Evans treat this topic more fully in the following chapter; hence only a few brief remarks will be made about the skill aspect of empathy here.

First, if empathy possesses a skill- or talent-like quality, it should have a genetic basis. Johnson, Cheek, and Smither (1983) suggest that this is indeed the case. Three of the four facets of empathy they identified (Social Self-Confidence, Even Temperedness, and Nonconformity) bear a close resemblance to three temperamental dispositions reported by Buss and Plomin (1975) to have significant heritability: Sociability, Emotionality, and Impulsivity.

Second, these genetic constraints will define how easy it will be to learn empathy and will place a limit on the degree to which one can improve one's empathic behavior. Anyone can learn, in theory, the footwork and movements involved in dunking a basketball, but only those with a given genetic endowment will actually be able to execute the dunk. So it is with empathy. To minimize trainee frustration in an empathy training program, realistic expectations should be tailored to individuals' potentials for empathic behavior.

A final comment concerns the age-old question of how an actor's "act" can be sincere or genuine. This question is particularly relevant to persons in the helping professions, for genuineness is generally regarded as an important element of the helping relationship (cf. Peitchinis, 1972). I suggested at the beginning of this chapter that genuineness is a function of the match between outer impressions and inner personality dispositions. A person who is not empathically motivated and/or lacks empathic skills can put on only a self-conscious, mechanical performance, which is perceived as phony by the audience. This is particularly true when the actor is "on stage" for long periods of time under demandingly high levels of stress—conditions that describe the typical hospital environment.

This is not to say that learning to go through the motions of empathy is pointless without the appropriate level of skill. To the degree that our *audience* is empathic, they will at least appreciate our attempt to be understanding and caring, even if our performances are somewhat clumsy. And, if we really care about others and truly desire to become skillfully empathic, this motive will support the long hours of practice necessary for developing genuine empathic skill.

REFERENCES

Allport, G. W. (1937). *Personality: A psychological interpretation*. New York: Holt, Rinehart and Winston.

Alston, W. P. (1975). Traits, consistency, and conceptual alternatives for personality theory. *Journal for the Theory of Social Behaviour, 5*, 17–48.

Baumeister, R. F. (Ed.) (1986). *Public self and private self*. New York: Springer-Verlag.

Block, J. (1961). *The Q-sort method in personality assessment and psychiatric research*. Springfield, IL: Charles C. Thomas.

Borman, W. C. (1979). Individual differences correlates of accuracy in evaluating others' performance effectiveness. *Applied Psychological Measurement, 3*, 103–115.

Bucheimer, A., & Balogh, S. C. (1961). *The counseling relationship: A casebook.* Chicago: Science Research Associates.

Buck, R., Miller, R. E., & Caul, W. F. (1974). Sex, personality, and physiological variables in the communication of emotion via facial expression. *Journal of Personality and Social Psychology, 30,* 587–596.

Buss, A. H., & Plomin, R. A. (1975). *A temperament theory of personality development.* New York: John Wiley.

D'Augelli, A. R. (1974). Nonverbal behavior of helpers in initial helping interactions. *Journal of Counseling Psychology, 21,* 360–363.

Ekman, P., (1965). Communication through nonverbal behavior. In S. S. Tomkins & C. E. Izard (Eds.), *Affect, cognition, and personality* (pp. 390–442). New York: Springer Publishing Company.

Ekman P., & Friesen, W. V. (1974). Detecting deception from the body or face. *Journal of Personality and Social Psychology, 29,* 288–298.

Exline, R. V., & Fehr, B. J. (1978). Applications of semiosis to the study of visual interaction. In A. W. Siegman & S. Feldstein (Eds.), *Nonverbal behavior and communication.* Hillsdale, NJ: Erlbaum.

Goffman, E. (1959). *The presentation of self in every day life.* New York: Doubleday Anchor Books.

Gough, H. G., & Heilbrun, A. B., Jr. (1965). *Manual for the Adjective Check List.* Palo Alto, CA: Consulting Psychologists Press.

Graves, J. R., & Robinson, J. D., II. (1976). Proxemic behavior as a function of inconsistent verbal and nonverbal messages. *Journal of Counseling Psychology, 23,* 333–338.

Heider, F. (1958). *The psychology of interpersonal relations.* New York: John Wiley.

Hendrick, C. (1977). Social psychology as an experimental science. In C. Hendrick (Ed.), *Perspectives on social psycholgy* (pp. 1–74). Hillsdale, NJ: Erlbaum.

Hogan, R. (1969). Development of an empathy scale. *Journal of Consulting and Clinical Psychology, 33,* 307–316.

Hogan, R. (1976). *Personality theory: The personological tradition.* Englewood Cliffs, NJ: Prentice-Hall.

Hogan, R. T. (1967). *Moral development: An assessment approach.* Unpublished doctoral dissertation, University of California, Berkeley.

Holland, J. L. (1985). *Making vocational choices* (2nd ed.). Englewood Cliffs, NJ: Prentice-Hall.

Johnson, J. A., Cheek, J. M., & Smither, R. (1983). The structure of empathy. *Journal of Personality and Social Psychology, 45,* 1299–1312.

Johnson, J. A., & Worley, L. D. (1987). Criminals' responses to religious themes in Whitman's poetry. In J. M. Day & W. S. Laufer (Eds.), *Crime, values, and religion* (pp. 133–151). Norwood, NJ: Ablex.

Kleinke, C. L. (1975). *First impressions: The psychology of encountering others.* Englewood Cliffs, NJ: Prentice-Hall.

Kraut, R. E. (1978). Verbal and nonverbal cues in the perception of lying. *Journal of Personality and Social Psychology, 36,* 380–391.

Kraut, R. E., & Johnston, R. E. (1979). Social and emotional messages of smiling: An ethological approach. *Journal of Personality and Social Psychology, 37*, 1539–53.

Kupfer, D. J., Drew, F. L., Curtis, E. K., & Rubinstein, D. N. (1978). Personality style and empathy in medical students. *Journal of Medical Education, 53*, 507–509.

La Monica, E. L. (1980, September). *Construct validity of an empathy instrument.* Paper presented at the 88th Annual Convention of the American Psychological Association, Montreal, Canada.

Lennenberg, E. H. (1967). *Biological foundations of language.* New York: John Wiley.

Lippa, R. (1978). Expressive control, expressive consistency, and the correspondence between expressive behavior and personality. *Journal of Personality, 46*, 438–461.

MacKinnon, D. W. (1944). The structure of personality. In J. McV. Hunt (Ed.), *Personality and the behavior disorders* (pp. 3–48). New York: Ronald Press.

Mills, C., & Hogan, R. (1978). A role theoretical interpretation of personality scale item responses. *Journal of Personality, 46*, 778–785.

Newman, B. M., & Newman, P. R. (1980). *Personality development through the life span.* Belmont, CA: Wadsworth.

Peitchinis, J. A. (1972). Therapeutic effectiveness of counseling by nursing personnel. *Nursing Research, 21*, 138–148.

Secord, P. F. (1958). Facial features and inference processes in interpersonal perception. In R. Tagiuri & L. Petrullo (Eds.), *Person perception and interpersonal behavior* (pp. 300–315). Stanford, CA: Stanford University Press.

Smith-Hanen, S. S. (1977). Effects of nonverbal behaviors on judged levels of counselor warmth and empathy. *Journal of Counseling Psychology, 24*, 420–429.

Tepper, D. T., Jr., & Haase, R. F. (1978). Verbal and nonverbal communication of facilitative conditions. *Journal of Counseling Psychology, 25*, 35–44.

5

Empathy as a Skill

George M. Gazda and Timothy D. Evans

Empathy is best defined at two levels. First, there is a conceptual definition of empathy as an attitude. Carl Rogers (1975) describes this as a way of being with another person. There is also an operational definition of empathy as a teachable communication skill. When Truax and Carkhuff (1967) researched Roger's concept of empathy, they made empathy into an observable behavior. By so doing they moved empathy away from being an attitude and made it into a teachable skill or a technology of communicating.

Gerard Egan's (1986) definition combines these two levels of empathy. He writes, "Empathy is the ability to enter into and understand the world of another person and communicate this understanding to him or her" (p. 95). Thus, a two-level definition best describes empathy as an attitude, and when operational, it is a communication skill.

EMPATHY AS AN ATTITUDE

Rogers (1975) maintained that empathy is an attitude and not a communication skill. He believed it is not so important what we say or do, but it is how we do it that makes us empathic. Rogers did not like the idea of empathy being translated into a technique of listening and reflecting feelings. He believed that empathy goes beyond listening, and it is an approach one assumes in relationship to another person. As a result of his concern, Rogers (1975) wrote:

The whole approach came, in a few years, to be known as a technique. "Nondirective therapy," it was said, "is a technique of reflecting the client's feelings". . . . I was so shocked by these complete distortions of our approach that for a number of years I said almost nothing about empathic listening, and when I did it was to stress an empathic attitude with little comment as to how this might be implemented in the relationship. (p. 3)

George Gazda's Human Relations Training (HRT) (Gazda, Asbury, Balzer, Childers, & Walters, 1984), now a part of his Life Skills Training (LST) model (Gazda, Childers, Brooks, 1987), teaches empathy as a skill. However, the HRT model also views empathy as an attitude. In fact, with HRT a respectful attitude is a prerequisite for obtaining the skills necessary for communicating empathic understanding.

HRT views this attitude in the context of psychosocial development. In order to obtain empathic skills, individuals must first reach a stage of development where they have a sincere interest in others. Developmentally, to be empathic individuals must have matured beyond thinking of themselves, so they are capable of understanding another's point of view.

All of us have this human potential to be interested in others, but this interest must be developed. Failure to develop this interest prevents us from being empathic, and leads to interpersonal difficulties. We might add, when HRT develops interpersonal skills it also facilitates the psychosocial development of the individual.

In the HRT model a respectful attitude means we trust human nature so much that we are comfortable allowing people to be themselves. This respect conveys belief in others' ability to solve their problems and correct their errors with minimum guidance. More specifically, a respectful attitude conveys that people are inherently worthwhile in spite of their differences, successes, and failures.

When we judge, control, and have expectations for others, we violate respect. Controlling, judging, and expecting the best from others conveys that people are not fine as they are. Instead, these attitudes tell people they need to do more or be more in order to be worthwhile.

Furthermore, when we lack respect we either do things *to* or *for* others but not *with* them. Doing things *to* or *for* others creates super-inferior relations which result in interpersonal conflicts. Anytime we do things to or for others we rob them of the experiences they need to develop into confident, self-reliant, and responsible human beings. Doing things for others, which they can do for themselves, not only handicaps them into dependency but conveys weakness in their ability to take care of themselves.

Along these lines HRT teaches that the facilitative helper conveys faith in persons to solve their own problems without giving advice. The facilitative helper responds with empathy and provides guidance when necessary. Guidance is working *with* people, offering encouragement, and freeing people to develop their own potential. Guidance maintains a respectful attitude by not interfering with the natural order of events. In contrast, advice-giving with its judging and controlling interferes with the natural order of events and obligates people to be a certain way. Advice-giving tells people what they should do, and this violates a respectful attitude.

EMPATHY AS A SKILL

To research Carl Rogers' core conditions of empathy, warmth, and genuineness, Truax and Carkhuff (1967) made these conditions into observable and measurable behaviors. They had to turn the core conditions into operational skills so they could be quantitatively measured. Thus, empathy moved from being an attitude, or a way of being, and became a concrete observable behavior that could be measured on the *Truax Accurate Empathy Scale* or the *Carkhuff Scales for Empathic Understanding* (Aspy, 1975). These scales allowed portions of recorded interviews to be used to reliably rate the level of empathy being conveyed by the helper. Truax developed an eight-point empathy scale while Carkhuff developed a five-point scale.

According to the Truax and Carkhuff scales, an empathic response is determined by how well we communicate understanding of a speaker's *feelings* and the *meaning* attached to those feelings. Failure to communicate this understanding means we either give a hurtful response, such as a put-down, or give a neutral *response* such as advice-giving. These low level responses were said to prevent a facilitative relationship from developing.

These two scales gave researchers not only a reliable instrument for rating responses but developed into human relations training models. Carkhuff used his scale not only for assessing classroom teachers, but developed it into a systematic approach for training professional service providers.

Carkhuff's model has been used to train educators (Gazda, et al., 1984), health care practitioners (Gazda, Childers, & Walters, 1982), and criminal justice personnel (Sisson, Arthur, & Gazda, 1981). Currently, there are similar programs such as *A Step Ahead In Caring* (Childers & Evans, 1987), that train empathy skills in health care professionals.

Thus, when Truax and Carkhuff translated empathy into an observable and measurable behavior, they shifted the definition away from Roger's empathic attitude and made it a communication *skill*. Bachrach (1976) comments that Carkhuff and Truax's scales changed Roger's idea of empathy from a way of being, which the helper assumes, into something the helper does.

MEANING WELL VS. DOING WELL

Many people mean well but they fail to do well because they lack the necessary skills. A sincere interest in others, without the skills to convey this interest, means we will not be perceived as empathic. Our meaning well will be sabotaged by our skill deficit.

In everyday situations, most of us attempt to convey our concern and understanding without the necessary skills. We limit the display of our concern by using overstocked phrases like, "I hear you," or "I understand." These responses are not necessarily hurtful, but they fail to convey understanding and do not communicate our caring attitude. In addition, most caring individuals at their very best respond with advice-giving. Unfortunately, this is the only response they know. When they give advice, they ignore what has been said and convey they are not really listening.

Childers and Evans (1987) found hospital employees reduce their professional effectiveness because they lack human relation skills. They have excellent technological skills but lack the necessary interpersonal skills needed to be effective. Without appropriate interpersonal skills, health-care professionals will be perceived by patients and others as not caring and lacking professionalism.

Today fewer medical personnel are getting by solely on their technological authority. To be perceived as professionally competent by the public, medical personnel need to be proficient in both their technological expertise and interpersonal skills.

Childers and Evans (1987) believe many hospital personnel *mean well* and care about patients, but there is disparity in their ability to *do well* interpersonally. They wrote:

> When a statement is made by a patient, visitor, or co-worker, the healthcare worker responds automatically without being sensitive to how the response is coming across to the other person. This can lead to situations where either hurtful or neutral responses are inadvertently given to others by well-meaning staff members. Hurtful responses are obvious, and both the employee and the other person will realize the interaction has been strained. (p. 29)

Meaning well versus having the skills to do well may further be explained by a patient's recent visit to a hospital's laboratory for a blood test. When the needle was placed in the patient's arm, the patient complained of a burning sensation. The technician responded, "Well, you have tough veins." This response was not hurtful but it certainly did not convey *understanding* of the patient's concern. It was a low level response. The technician may have meant well, but she lacked the interpersonal skills necessary to communicate her understanding. In addition, the patient perceived the technician, along with the hospital, as incompetent.

The technician would have appeared understanding and professionally competent if she gave an empathic response. For example, if she had said, "You're feeling discomfort from the needle," or "Your arm is hurting more than you think it should," the patient would have felt understood and respected by the technician. Instead, he felt misunderstood and not cared for by the technician.

In summary, a definition of empathy needs to include a discussion of empathy as an attitude and a skill. By doing both, we can mean well *and* do well; otherwise, we will be like the lab technician. We will know our jobs and care about patients but lack the skills necessary to convey this caring. Yet on the other hand, to have the technology of communicating understanding and to lack the necessary attitude will make us mechanical and unfeeling. In order for empathy to occur, we need to master both the attitudes and skills.

EMPATHY: A TEACHABLE SKILL

There is substantial evidence that suggests empathy is an essential, if not a necessary, ingredient for effective learning to occur. There is solid evidence that shows in counseling and education that empathic relationships lead to significant improvement in client functioning and student performance. In addition, Aspy (1975) has shown that professionals like doctors, lawyers, and even prison guards function at low empathic levels and would improve their effectiveness if they received human relations training.

Aspy believes empathy is essential for positive human development, and it needs to be taught to everyone. He thinks our entire society would benefit from learning the application of empathy to human relations. Aspy recommends that empathy training be a part of every service-oriented profession. Unfortunately, most professions leave the ability to be empathic to chance. Consequently, some have it, while most do not.

Rogers, Truax, Carkhuff, and Gazda all believe empathy is a human potential which must be developed and not left to chance. Rogers, however, differs in how empathy should be developed. He thinks empathy is best taught by being around other empathic persons. Rogers believes the empathic *climate* itself, teaches others to be empathic, while those who view empathy as more than an attitude, suggest it be directly taught as a skill like other skills are taught in school.

Gazda's HRT model recommends empathy be taught as one teaches the rules of grammar (Gazda, et al., 1987):

> Individuals can learn effective components of interpersonal communication/human relations in a fashion similar to the ways they learn the rules of grammar and speaking. If we take into account the person's developmental level and readiness to learn, the concepts of the model can then be taught with increasing degrees of complexity to children, adolescents, and adults by using the coping skill and developmental tasks descriptors. (pp. 177–178)

There is agreement among all the authors mentioned that the degree of empathy we posses correlates with our personal development. In other words, the level at which we learn and are empathic coexists with our level of functioning. Rogers (1975) best describes this view when he wrote:

> The better integrated the therapist is within himself, the higher degree of empathy he exhibits . . . I come to the somewhat uncomfortable conclusion that the more psychologically mature and integrated the therapist is as a person, the more helpful is the relationship he provides. (p. 5)

The HRT model describes this same concept but in terms of psychosocial development. In HRT terms, if we are not able to view life from another person's perspective, then we cannot be empathic. Failure to master specific psychosocial tasks means developmentally we are not capable of empathy.

Training models, like HRT, are advantageous because they are used to develop skills and remedy psychosocial development. For instance, HRT matches the level of skills with the level of development found in the individual. As individuals master specific skills and function at higher levels interpersonally, they advance in their psychosocial development. By remedying deficiencies in basic human relation skills, individuals not only learn how to be empathic, but they are able to develop psychosocially.

The HRT model attempts to teach empathy throughout our lifetime. With each stage of psychosocial development, beginning with childhood, basic empathy skills can be taught. As we master one developmental stage we are able to advance to the next level of interpersonal functioning. Thus, the HRT skills help advance us developmentally from adolescence through adulthood.

In summary, the HRT model offers skills that can be used both for remedial training and for prevention of skill deficits. With HRT we begin to learn empathic attitudes and skills at their most teachable moment and progress according to our psychosocial development. This allows us to learn the necessary skills needed for our interpersonal functioning. It also allows us to avoid difficulties that could appear in our development because we lack basic interpersonal skills.

LIFE SKILLS TRAINING AND EMPATHY SKILLS

HRT is a part of Gazda's Life Skills Training (LST) and makes up the generic life-skill interpersonal communication/human relations. Besides interpersonal communication/human relations, there are three other generic life-skills: problem solving/decision making, physical fitness/health maintenance, and identity development/purpose in life.

The LST model is designed for prevention, as well as to remedy problems, with mastery of the generic life-skill interpersonal communication/human relations a prerequisite to learning the other three. This section will describe teaching empathy as a skill to health care professionals using the HRT model found in Gazda's LST.

The HRT model uses a group format in teaching empathy. The training requires a minimum of 12 group hours. The optimal group size ranges between 10 to 18 members. Most trainers prefer a group consisting of 12 members. A major function of the group is to allow trainees the opportunity to practice the skills they are learning. With each skill component there are exercises that allow group members to practice and successfully master the skills. Once a skill is mastered, group members move on to the more advanced skills.

The HRT consists of three major skills: (1) recognizing and classifying types of requests, (2) attending behaviors, and (3) giving empathic responses. These three areas will be outlined below.

The first set of empathy skills to be mastered in the group setting is recognizing and classifying types of requests. In a medical setting, one must be able to assess if a patient is making an interpersonal or professional request. Technically, a patient can make four kinds of requests to a health care professional. Each request requires a different response from the health care provider.

The first two requests, *request for information* and *request for action*, involve professional or technical expertise. These requests do not involve interpersonal concerns and are the easiest to manage. The patient either asks for some appropriate and basic information or action. A request for information may be, "What time do I see the doctor tomorrow?" This request asks for information. A request for action asks you to do something such as, "Please hand me a glass of water."

The third request, *request for understanding and involvement*, requires the greatest skill in interpersonal functioning. A request for understanding and involvement deals with a patient's personal concerns versus a professional or technical concern. It requires the health care provider to convey empathic understanding. Frequently these requests are misperceived and treated as requests for information or action. When this occurs, the individual is given advice or told what to do instead of being understood.

A statement such as, "I am really worried about tomorrow and don't think I can sleep tonight," is a request for understanding. It is to be met with an empathic response. Advice such as, "Well, talk to your physician about getting a sleeping pill," is not hurtful but it shows little understanding. The HRT model focuses on how to give an empathic response to such a request.

The fourth type of request an employee may encounter is an *inappropriate request*. These requests attempt to engage the health care provider in gossip, breaching confidentiality, or participating in unethical behavior. They are to be met with firm, yet friendly behavior which conveys the message, "I do not engage in this type of behavior" (Childers & Evans, 1987).

Upon mastery of identifying these different forms of requests, group members advance to learning attending skills. These are nonverbal behaviors used for listening to another person. These behaviors include tone of voice, posture, eye contact, facial expressions, and other physical behaviors.

Effective attending skills nonverbally convey interest in the other person. Attending behaviors communicate a willingness to give others your time and attention. By attending, you make it easier for the patients to discuss the personal difficulty they are experiencing.

Think how difficult it is to develop a conversation while someone is looking at their watch, fixing their hair, glancing around the room, or in a hurry as you attempt to talk. It is highly unlikely that a facilitative relationship will develop when someone acts distracted and disinterested in what you are saying. Attending skills let the speaker know you are interested in hearing what he or she has to say.

Upon mastery of attending skills, group members are ready to develop the ability to give *facilitative responses*. These responses are used when a request for understanding/involvement is made by the patient. Facilitative responses require one to have proficient attending skills, so nonverbally they can convey empathic understanding.

A facilitative response is one that accurately perceives the speaker's feelings and conveys that understanding to the speaker. These responses can be measured for their empathic content on the *Empathy Scale* shown in Table 5.1 (Gazda, et al., 1984).

The *Empathy Scale* is a seven-point scale with 3.0 being a facilitative response. A 1.0 to 2.5 response does not convey understanding and respect for an individual. These responses range from a hurtful to a neutral response. Whereas, a 3.0, 3.5, or 4.0 response is empathic, conveys respect, and forms a facilitative relationship.

Before learning how to give a 3.5 or 4.0 response, group members learn how to give a basic 3.0 facilitative response. Defined by the Empathy Scale, a 3.0 response is one which communicates the primary *feelings* made by the helpee and includes the *meaning* the helpee attaches to these feelings. In essence, a 3.0 response conveys understanding of how the helpee feels (affect) and the meaning (content) attached to those feelings.

The first step in giving an empathic response is to listen carefully and determine if the helpee is making a request for understanding. If so, the next step is to determine what words represent the helpee's affect and content. The final step is stating your understanding to the helpee in an empathic statement that conveys the helpee's affect and content.

To illustrate, suppose a patient states, "Being in the hospital today means I missed my grandson's birthday." A 3.0 response would accurately perceive the patient's surface feeling (disappointment) and content (missed birthday). Placed in a sentence it would look like this, "You are disappointed because you missed a very special occasion."

The statement is technologically sound and earns a 3.0 on the *Empathy Scale*. However, empathy is an art regardless of how technologically accurate we become. If this statement is made with the appropriate attitude and the patient perceives you as understanding, then you gave an empathic response.

The statement given may seem simple, yet it takes a concentrated effort since our usual tendency is to give advice or change the focus from the helpee to ourselves. A simple exercise is to observe how often during a day you really listen to someone and convey your understanding of what was said. In practice, many of us find it difficult to really listen and convey our understanding. We all have the tendency to give advice, change the subject, or solve the other person's problem since this takes less time.

Finally, a three-phase cycle of problem solving is developed from giving facilitative responses with empathy being at the core of this cycle. These three phases are: (1) *self-exploration*, (2) *self-understanding*, and (3) *action*.

Briefly stated, self-exploration is when patients have a "fuzzy mess" and begin to explore their feelings, behaviors, and experiences relevant to their problems. The skills needed for self-exploration are the basic 3.0 empathic response skills.

Self-exploration leads patients into the next phase of self-understanding. Here the problem is defined in more concrete terms. In this phase, empathy, along with specific skills, such as immediacy, appropriate self-disclosure, genuineness, and 3.5 empathic responses is used.

Table 5.1 Empathy Scale

1.0	1.5	2.0	2.5	3.0	3.5	4.0
An irrelevant hurtful response that does not appropriately attend to the surface feelings of the helpee. However, in instances where content is communicated accurately, it may raise the level of the response.		A response that only partially communicates an awareness of the surface feelings of the helpee. When content is communicated accurately it may raise the level of response; conversely, it may lower the level of the response when communicated inaccurately.		A response conveying that the helpee is understood at the level he or she is expressing; surface feelings are accurately reflected. Content is not essential, but, when included, it must be accurate. If it is inaccurate, level of the response may be lowered.		A response conveying that the helpee is understood beyond his or her level of immediate awareness; underlying feelings are identified. Content is used to complement affect in adding deeper meaning. If content is inaccurate, the level of the response may be lowered.

Keywords—Empathy Scale
Level 4.0—underlying feelings; additive
Level 3.0—surface feelings reflected
Level 2.0—subtractive
Level 1.0—irrelevant; hurtful

Reprinted by permission from *Human relations development: A manual for educators* (3rd ed.) G. M. Gazda, F. Asbury, F. J. Blazer, W. C. Childers, and R. P. Walters. Boston: Allyn and Bacon, Inc., 1984, p. 88.

Once the problem is defined in concrete terms during the self-understanding phase, patients are ready for the action phase. In this phase patients begin to develop a plan of action for solving their problems. This stage relies on empathic understanding but also uses such skills as appropriate confrontation and setting behavioral goals (Egan, 1975, 1986).

SUMMARY

Empathy, viewed as both an attitude and a skill, bridges the disparity between meaning well and doing well. Developing the skills necessary to communicate empathy allows us to convey our caring attitude. These skills must be developed and practiced in a learning environment. Without such skills training, communicating our empathic attitude is left to chance and usually results in advice-giving instead of communicating understanding.

This chapter gave an overview of empathy as an attitude and when operational as a communication skill. A rationale for providing HRT has been given along with the group format used to teach empathy skills.

REFERENCES

Aspy, D. N. (1975). Empathy: Let's get the hell on with it. *The Counseling Psychologist, 5,* (2), 10–14.

Bachrach, M. B. (1976). Empathy. *Archives of General Psychiatry, 33,* 35–38.

Childers, W. C., & Evans, T. D. (1987). The interpersonal environment. *Administrative Radiology, 6*(2), 29–33.

Egan, G. (1975). *The skilled helper.* California: Wadsworth Publishing Company.

Egan, G. (1986). *The skilled helper.* California: Brooks Cole Publishing Company.

Gazda, G. M., Childers, W. C., Walters, R. P., (1982). *Interpersonal Communications.* Rockville, MD: Aspen Publication.

Gazda, G. M., Asbury, F. S., Balzer, F. J., Childers, W. C., & Walters, R. P., (1984). *Human relations development.* Boston: Allyn and Bacon Inc.

Gazda, G. M., Childers, W. C., & Brooks, D. K., Jr., (1987). *Foundations of counseling and human services.* New York: McGraw-Hill.

Rogers, C. R. (1957). The necessary and sufficient conditions of therapeutic personality change. *Journal of Consulting Psychology, 21,* 95–103.

Rogers, C. R. (1975). Empathic: an unappreciated way of being. *The Counseling Psychologist, 5,* (2), 2–9.

Truax, C. B., & Carkhuff, R. R. (1967). *Toward effective counseling and psychotherapy.* Chicago: Aldine.

6

A Model of Empathy
in the Helping Relationship

Ruth C. MacKay
Jean R. Hughes
E. Joyce Carver

A MODEL OF EMPATHY
IN THE HELPING RELATIONSHIP

In this chapter we put forward a conceptual model to facilitate examination of the professional's use of empathy, along with its consequences, in professional–client interaction. Components of the model introduced and discussed in earlier chapters are reviewed, in relation to the dynamic quality of the interaction process, and within the context of environmental constraints.

THE EMPATHIC PROFESSIONAL

Professionals vary in their abilities to offer empathy in a helping relationship (Carkhuff, 1969; Gazda, Walters, & Childers, 1975; La Monica, Carew, Winder, Haase, & Blanchard, 1976; Layton, 1979; Peitchinis, 1976; Traux & Carkhuff, 1967). Previous chapters suggest that the ability to be empathic can be derived from two sources: personality disposition and learned ability.

Influences of Personal Characteristics

Not unexpectedly, personal characteristics of the helping professional may exert influences on the interaction process. These characteristics can be classed as biological, psychological, and
socio-cultural.

Biological characteristics

The influence of the professional's age, gender, race, and other
biological attributes may modify empathy in a helping relationship.
However, the effects of these variables are as yet undocumented,
or studies have shown conflicting results. For example, Mynatt
(1985) stated that age and sex did not correlate with empathy and
Nagel (1984/1985) reported age to be a nonsignificant factor. In
contrast, Pennington (1981) found sex and age to be significant
predictors in explaining nursing home personnel's empathy toward
the aged, and Steibe, Boulet, and Lee (1979) indicated age affected
successful training in empathic functioning of Roman Catholic
nuns who were non-professional counselors.

Psychological characteristics

There are a number of personality factors that have been studied
in relation to empathy; altruism, humanitarianism, and dogmatism
are examples (See Batson, O'Quin, Fultz, Vanderplas, & Isen, 1983;
Collins, 1972; Streit-Forest, 1982, Toi & Batson, 1982). Empathy
itself is also viewed as a personality disposition affecting the
professional's ability to be therapeutic while interacting with a
client. Johnson has discussed dispositional empathy in detail in
Chapter 4.

Cultural and social influences

Sociocultural factors have been linked to empathy. Suar (1982/1984)
found the interaction of tribal status and gender affected the empathy of college students in India. Watson, Hood, Morris, and Hall
(1984) reported that religiosity was related to empathy. In addition,
education, professional or work experience, and social class have
been studied in relation to empathy (see Bath & Calhoun, 1977;
Diseker & Michielutte, 1981; Mullen & Abeles, 1971; Mynatt, 1985;
and Pennington, 1981). Davis discusses culture in relation to empathy in professional–client practice in Chapter 11.

Perception of role

Norms of behavior govern any interaction process. The professional is influenced by prescriptions which dictate the realm and standards of practice, the specific focus of clinical attention, ethics, and what constitutes "good" behavior in the eyes of professional peers. Hills and Knowles (1983) suggest "that interpersonal skills in nursing have been learned in psychiatric settings and are considered to be applicable primarily in those settings" (p. 87). They identify the need to alter role expectations for facilitative interaction in all settings. Hogan sees the empathic person as able to adjust role in relation to the perception of impression made on the other person in the interaction (1975, p. 15). This suggests that role expectations can be important modifiers of perceived empathy.

Empathy Skill

The professional's skill in the use of empathy has been noted to be a strong determinant of how empathy is manifested in professional–client interaction. Programs to educate helping professionals in the use of empathy have been successful in raising the level of facilitative empathy in client encounters. This supports the view that the use of empathy is a learned skill. This approach has been discussed in detail by Gazda and Evans in Chapter 5.

THE CLIENT IN NEED

The presenting characteristics of the client are important in the interaction process as well as those of the professional. However, few studies were found reporting the influence of these variables. Stotland, Sherman, and Kelly (1971) and Barbarin and Chesler (1984) note that when clients are seen by professionals as being similar to themselves the professionals show more empathy. This relationship is modified by birth order in respect to the professionals. On the other hand, Wasserman, Inui, Barriatua, Carter, and Lippincott (1984/1985) found that the observed level of empathy of pediatric clinicians was not related to demographic factors of mothers of infants.

The dependency of clients has received attention. Hardin and

Halaris (1983) attributed specific observed nonverbal behaviors in nurse–patient interaction, such as torso-moving, laughter, and eye contact, to a dependent or subordinant client role (p. 15). Gagan in 1983 commented that the passive dependent role of the client could account for Forsyth's finding that clients perceive all nurses as empathic, whether they are or not as shown by objective evidence (p. 70). This passive role was the expected norm for client behavior until the emergence of the self-help and consumer movements in health care which call for greater participation in health-related decision making and for control over one's own body and life. Barbarin and Chesler (1984/1985) noted that parents of children with cancer perceived medical staff members more positively when empathy with the child was seen to be high. The role was characterized as one of positive personal contact.

Factors related to the client's presenting problem also may have a bearing on the professional's mobilization of empathy skills in professional–client interaction. The urgency of acute situations may narrow the professional's attention to immediate interventions, with interpersonal interaction taking on secondary importance. Furthermore, the treatment regimen may modify interaction so that the use of empathy is obscured or deterred, for example, when face masks are worn by the helping professionals, or the patient is receiving respiratory assistance by means of a mechanical ventilator. In addition, attribution theory suggests that patients who are victims of accidents have been blamed by professionals (and others) for having invited the occurrence through negative behaviors, such as negligence or carelessness. (See Damrosch, 1985 and Lerner, 1980.)

In summary, there are a number of situational factors or characteristics stemming from the client which may influence the professional in offering empathy.

ENVIRONMENTAL INFLUENCES AFFECTING INTERACTION

The physical, social, cultural, and emotional environments affect professional–client interaction in a number of ways. In addition, temporal constraints may inflict rather severe restrictions on the interacting pair.

Physical Factors

Physical space has been found to influence social interaction. Hall (1966), for example, described the qualities of communication in terms of differing distances between the interacting pair. Closer proximities supported more personal communication. The relationship may be curvilinear, however, in professional–client interaction, because helping professionals who must enter the client's private space to give treatment bring into play a number of ploys to give distance to offset the effects of unwanted otherwise-perceived intimacy, ploys such as cessation of eye contact.

Privacy, noise, and room temperature obviously affect communication as well. The type of setting is a factor which Pennington (1981) noted has influenced observed empathy. He reported that profit institutions (nursing homes) exerted greater influence on empathy of staff than did non-profit institutions. Brunt (1985), however, found that nurses using technological equipment in hospital intensive care areas are not, as hypothesized, less empathic than those who work in non-intensive care areas. The relationship between the physical environment and the professional's perceived empathy is obviously complex, and not yet fully explored.

Emotional Climate

It can be expected that factors from the emotional environment of the situation in which interaction takes place can influence the way professionals use empathy. For example, organizational factors, such as the time clients wait for attention in a clinic visit, may be a source of stress. Other stressors could be the consideration of health care costs, the tempo of activity in an office or health care unit, and interruptions during the interaction period. Factors such as these, recognized or not, may affect the emotional climate of the interaction situation and should be included in a conceptual model examining empathy in professional practice.

Norms Governing Relationships

There are numerous norms stemming from the social and cultural environment which dictate behavior in a professional–client relationship. Norms cover areas of practice such as confidentiality of information disclosed and expectations for compliance with recommended treatment. Symmetry in the relationship is another example. There is the expectation that the professional will reach out to the client to enable the client to discuss the presenting problem for which help is sought. This requires the client to reveal personal information. However, the professional is not expected to reciprocate by divulging information which is related to the professional's personal problems. The relationship is asymmetrical in order to keep the focus of attention on the client. Merton and Barber (1963) have identified a number of norms which govern interaction in medical practice and they described ambivalence in the way in which these norms may be perceived.

Peitchinis (1976) has noted the need to consider how health practices recommended by professionals may conflict with norms and values held by individuals from particular subcultures (p. 7). How does the professional's knowledge of cultural values enhance or inhibit empathy in professional–client interaction? This is discussed by Davis in Chapter 11 and is a variable to include in a model of empathy.

Temporal Constraints

Timing in the interaction is of importance to both professional and client. Whereas the professional may be concerned with fleeting time and the flow of tasks to be accomplished in a busy day, the client's attention may be more focused on the moment. What are the effects on empathic communication? Forsyth (1980) states that "the 'here and now' experience is important and must be responded to; otherwise changes occur in time and space" (p. 35). New feelings and thoughts replace past experience if the moment is lost to postponement.

A number of factors from the physical, social, cultural, and emotional environments in which professional–client interaction transpires have been discussed. These environmental variables, along with time constraints, exert powerful influences on professional–client interaction.

EMPATHY IN THE COMMUNICATION PROCESS

We have discussed variables which may influence empathy in professional–client communication from the perspective of what the professional, the client, and the environment contribute. However, the combination of factors from these sources in the interaction process adds other influences to the system under study which serve to modify outcome behaviors. For example, although helping professionals may have skill in the use of empathy, cues from the client's situation may make salient the professional's psychological disposition to offer help. Observations from laboratory and field experiments support the finding that professionals may act from egoistic as well as altruistic motivations, and interpretation of client need depends to a large extent on the perception of the entire presenting situation. (See Batson et al., 1983; Betancourt, 1983; Coke, Batson, & McDavis, 1978; Toi & Batson, 1982, and the discussion of these factors by Johnson in Chapter 4). Futhermore, the client's processing of received empathy influences the interpretation of the professional's message, based on numerous variables, such as past experience and cultural values (see Chapter 11 for Davis' discussion of cultural factors). Moreover, the professional processes the client's responses as well, and the meaning inferred may influence the use of empathy in ensuing interchanges. In illustration, the professional's need to protect self when the interaction poses threatening consequences may cause the professional to withdraw from the interaction, either physically or psychologically (see Stotland, Mathews, Sherman, Hansson, & Richardson (1978) for a full discussion of this behavior).

The interaction process is obviously dynamic, continually producing new stimuli for both professional and client to assimilate as the interaction proceeds. Communication may change in scope or direction or both, and move between facilitating, or inhibiting, the achievement of outcomes pertinent to the client's wellbeing. We use the Gage (Avis, Drysdale, Gregg, Neufeldt, & Scargill, 1983) dictionary definition of "wellbeing" as "health and happiness" (p. 1277), a term which in our view is quite similar to Dunn's (1959) meaning of "wellness." Not only can interaction be classed as neutral, positive, or negative in moving the client towards increased wellbeing, but the effects can be cumulative over succeeding encounters, or as the client communicates with one helping professional after another. What is the effect, for example, on perceived empathy if the client brings a stereotyping process into play in storing impressions from past encounters? Thus the affect from the interactions may not be extinguished at the termination of the exchange. How do such encounters move transitory feelings into more stable attitudes? These questions need study.

A MODEL OF EMPATHY
IN PROFESSIONAL–CLIENT INTERACTION

We have examined empathy in a helping relationship, noting that the interactive effects of factors in the professional–client encounter may modify how empathy is perceived and how it is offered. It is important now to consider in our model how empathy affects client outcomes. Client self–disclosures are one immediate consequence of the professional's use of empathy, and this is discussed in Chapter 9. Client feelings, that is, transitory emotional reactions, towards the professional and the health care or other agency, and the client's view of self, may be affected additionally by the professional's use of empathy. These may be seen as immediate outcomes because they are more directly related to the current interaction situation. The continuing effects of the professional's use of empathy on client attitudes and wellbeing can be expected to follow, but these effects are difficult to attribute only to the influence of empathy. The treatment program, or competing demands for the client's attention, energy, and other resources, among many things, may impinge on the relationship of empathy to the selected outcome, obscuring the observation of significant effects. Yet these problems may result not so much from difficulty in formulating a multivariable theoretical explanation of empathy in professional–client interaction, but from the inability to fully operationalize outcomes to gain precise measurement of effects.

We developed a model of empathy in professional–client interaction to assist us to examine various contributing factors related to the operation of empathy in a practice setting. The model represents dyadic interaction and is depicted in Figure 6.1. With the introduction of other health team members, or perhaps the client's family, into the interaction situation, the model could be expanded to incorporate this added complexity. However, our research has been limited to analysis of one-to-one relationships only. Some research has been cited in support of particular conceptual linkages. A number of these linkages are discussed in previous chapters and in those that follow.

An example is given to illustrate the enactment of empathy, and its consequences, in a professional–client exchange during a treatment procedure. A nurse is changing the dressings on two leg wounds of a patient hospitalized for burns. Just prior to the pa-

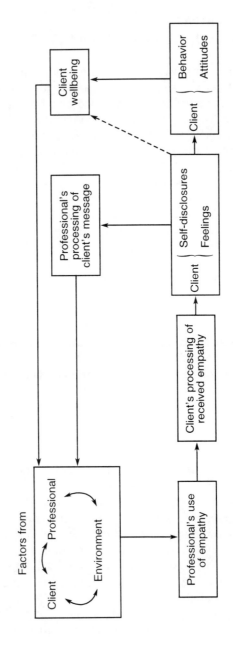

FIGURE 6.1 A model of empathy in professional-client interaction.

tient's accident the patient was interviewed for a new job. He heard later that he was to be hired. Treatment for the burns he had sustained was estimated to take about eight weeks. The patient in previous encounters with the nurse had expressed his feelings of elation in winning the position over other candidates. This elation was marred, however, by his anxiety over the uncertainty of being able to retain the job opportunity by reason of his lengthy hospitalization. This is the situation when the nurse on a particular day began the dressing change.

> N: Where shall we begin? (and when this was indicated) Do you want to take the old dressing off yourself?
> P: Yes. I'm glad you let me help. It hurts less. I'll take it off here first.
> N: I can see it's very painful for you, but this way you can tell yourself when you're ready.
> P: You know, if I can do this much, maybe I can learn to do the whole dressing myself, and I won't be in here so long after all. Maybe I'll be able to hold that new job in spite of everything.

The nurse demonstrated empathy in overtly recognizing the patient's pain. Allowing the patient control over the timing of the painful procedure showed the nurse's respect for the patient as well as his ability to manage his pain. These might be the impressions the patient is processing as a result of the nurse's statement, facilitating his following decision to reveal more of his thoughts, about his future, tentatively trying out the idea "I'm in control of my situation today, why not later? Why couldn't I be ready for my new job?" These feelings may have bolstered his self-confidence, supporting a positive outlook to his vocational future, moving him towards a feeling of wellbeing. The nurse also processes the information the patient has offered and can use it in the repetition of the cycle in subsequent exchanges.

In our own research, described in Part Three, we address three particular areas of the model, that of the effects of the professional's use of empathy on (a) client self-disclosures (b) expressed client concerns, and (c) the process of the professional-client interaction. The model should be viewed as a beginning attempt to depict the factors and interrelationships involved in the complex phenomenon of empathy in professional–client interaction. Therefore it is undoubtedly incomplete.

SUMMARY

This chapter has discussed various factors affecting observed empathy of professionals while in interaction with their clients. Factors stemming from the professional, the client, the interactional environment, and the interrelationships of these factors, are put forward in a model to explain empathy and its immediate and more long-term effects on client wellbeing. Subsequent chapters discuss the testing of segments of the model with implications for adjustment of the model and further research.

REFERENCES

Avis, W. S., Drysdale, P. D., Gregg, R. J., Neufeldt, V. E., & Scargill, M. H. (1983). *Gage Canadian Dictionary.* Toronto: Gage Educational Publishing.

Barbarin, O. A., & Chesler, M. A. (1984). Relationships with the medical staff and aspects of satisfaction with care expressed by parents of children with cancer. *Journal of Community Health, 9*(4), 302–313. (From *Medline Abstracts,* 1985, No. 85007568)

Bath, K. E., & Calhoun, R. O. (1977). The effects of professional counselor training on empathy: Continued cause for concern. *Counselor Education and Supervision, 17*(2), 98–106.

Batson, C. D., O'Quin, K., Fultz, J., Vanderplas, M., & Isen, A. M. (1983). Influence of self-reported distress and empathy on egoistic versus altruistic motivation to help. *Journal of Personality and Social Psychology, 45,* 706–718.

Betancourt, H. (1983). Causal attributions, empathy, and emotions as determinants of helping behavior: An integrative approach. *Dissertation Abstracts International, 44,* 1636B.

Brunt, J. H. (1985). An exploration of the relationship between nurses' empathy and technology. *Nursing Administration Quarterly, 9*(4), 69–78.

Carkhuff, R. R. (1969). *Helping and human relations: A primer for lay and professional helpers.* Vols. 1 & 2. New York: Holt, Rinehart, & Winston.

Coke, J. S., Batson, C. D., & McDavis, K. (1978). Empathic mediation of helping: A two-stage model. *Journal of Personality and Social Psychology, 36,* 752–766.

Collins, D. L. (1972). Empathic ability and dogmatism in nursing students (Doctoral dissertation, Teachers College, Columbia University, 1972). *Dissertation Abstracts International, 33,* 2609A.

Damrosch, S. P. (1985). Nursing students' assessments of behaviorally self-blaming rape victims. *Nursing Research, 34,* 221–224.

Diseker, R. A., & Michielutte, R. (1981). An analysis of empathy in medical students before and following clinical experience. *Journal of Medical Education, 56*, 1004–1010.

Forsyth, G. L. (1980). Analysis of the concept of empathy: Illustration of one approach. *Advances in Nursing Science, 2*(2), 33–42.

Gagan, J. M. (1983). Methodological notes on empathy. *Advances in Nursing Science, 5*(2), 65–72.

Gazda, G. M., Walters, R. P., & Childers, W. C. (1975). *Human relations development: A manual for health sciences.* Boston: Allyn & Bacon.

Hall, E. (1966). *The hidden dimension.* New York: Doubleday.

Hardin, S. B., & Halaris, A. L. (1983). Nonverbal communication of patients and high and low empathy nurses. *Journal of Psychosocial Nursing and Mental Health Services, 21*(1), 14–20.

Hills, M. D., & Knowles, D. (1983). Nurses' levels of empathy and respect in simulated interactions with patients. *International Journal of Nursing Studies, 20*(2), 83–87.

Hogan, R. (1975). Empathy: A conceptual and psychometric analysis. *The Counseling Psychologist, 5*(2), 14–18.

La Monica, E. L., Carew, D. K., Winder, A. E., Haase, A. M. B., & Blanchard, K. H. (1976). Empathy training as the major thrust of a staff development program. *Nursing Research, 25*, 447–451.

Layton, J. M. (1979). The use of modeling to teach empathy to nursing students. *Research in Nursing and Health, 2*, 163–176.

Lerner, M. J. (1980). *The belief in a just world.* New York: Plenum.

Merton, R. K., & Barber, E. (1963). Sociological ambivalence. In E. A. Tiryakian (Ed.). *Sociological theory, values, and sociocultural change* (pp. 91–120). New York: Free Press.

Mullen, J., & Abeles, N. (1971). Relationship of liking, empathy, and therapist's experience to outcome of therapy. *Journal of Consulting Psychology, 18*(1), 39–43.

Mynatt, S. (1985). Empathy in faculty and students in different types of nursing preparation programs. *Western Journal of Nursing Research, 7*, 333–348.

Nagel, J. (1984/1985). Facilitative effectiveness of elderly and adolescent volunteer counselors in a nursing home setting. *Dissertation Abstracts International, 45*, 3953B.

Peitchinis, J. A. (1976). *Staff–patient communication in the health services.* New York: Springer Publishing Co.

Pennington, R. E. (1981). An observational study of empathy and selected variables in New Orleans nursing homes with implications for the development of in-service training programs. *Dissertation Abstracts International, 42*, 2245A.

Steibe, S. C., Boulet, D. B., & Lee, D. C. (1979). Trainee trait empathy, age, trainer functioning, client age and training time as discriminators of successful empathy training. *Canadian Counsellor, 14*(1), 41–46.

Stotland, E., Mathews, K. E., Jr., Sherman, S. E., Hansson, R. O., & Richardson, B. Z. (1978). *Empathy, fantasy, and helping*. Beverly Hills: Sage.

Stotland, E., Sherman, S. E., & Shaver, K. G. (1971). *Empathy and birth order*. Lincoln: University of Nebraska Press.

Streit-Forest, U. (1982). Differences in empathy: A preliminary analysis. *Journal of Medical Education, 57*(1), 65–67.

Suar, D. (1982). Role of tribal, non tribal status, sex and academic achievement on empathy. *Indian Psychological Review, 22*(2), 11–15. (From *Psychological Abstracts*, 1984, 71, Abstract No. 4041).

Toi, M., & Batson, C. D. (1982). More evidence that empathy is a source of altruistic motivation. *Journal of Personality and Social Psychology, 43*, 281–292.

Truax, C. B., & Carkhuff, R. R. (1967). *Toward effective counseling and psychotherapy: Training and practice*. Chicago: Aldine.

Wasserman, R. C., Inui, T. S., Barriatua, R. D., Carter, W. B., & Lippincott, P. (1984). Pediatric clinicians' support for parents makes a difference: An outcome-based analysis of clinician–parent interaction. *Pediatrics, 74*, 1047–1053. (From *Medline Abstracts*, 1985 No. 85062674).

Watson, P. J., Hood, R. W., Jr., Morris, R. J., & Hall, J. R. (1984). Empathy, religious orientation, and social desirability. *The Journal of Psychology, 117*, 211–216.

7

The Measurement
of Empathy

Ruth C. MacKay
Jean R. Hughes
E. Joyce Carver

The measurement of empathy as a component of professional-client interaction serves two purposes: (a) to measure the ability of professionals to offer empathy as part of an assessment of clinical competence, and (b) to investigate the use of empathy and its influence on client wellbeing. In the past, investigators have used a variety of approaches to measure empathy. Each of these measurement approaches stems from a different view of empathy as a concept: from a behavioral orientation, as a dimension of personality, and as experienced emotions engendered when observing the emotions of others. See Chapter 1 for a description of three basic ways in which empathy is conceptualized, as revealed in the published literature.

Operationalizing the different concepts of empathy from an abstract to a concrete form has led to further variations in empathy as a construct. This has direct influence in the measurement process. This chapter examines basic conceptualizations of empathy in terms of the constructs drawn from them, with examples of the measuring instruments which have been reported, as relevant to each. Instruments are categorized as relying on: (a) observer ratings, (b) client perceptions, (c) professionals' self-ratings, (d) peer ratings, (e) tests inferring ability to offer empathy, (f) personality measures, (g) experimental manipulation of enacted empathy to study the observer's response, and (h) tests to assess the experienced emotion of the observer in a situation created to invoke empathy. Conclusions are drawn as they relate to clinical practice and research. The accurate and valid measurement of empathy is a formidable research goal not yet fully achieved. Without a dependable measure, research cannot proceed in the testing of hypotheses concerning the impact of the professional's use of empathy on client outcomes.

EMPATHY AS A CONSTRUCT

Researchers vary in how they make the concept of empathy concrete. The different constructs which emerge reflect the central focus of one particular component of the concept. Loosely these fall into the three major categories of empathy as a behavior, as a personality dimension, and as experienced emotion.

MEASUREMENT OF EMPATHIC BEHAVIOR

Behavior indicative of the professional's use of empathy can be judged by an independent observer, or by those involved in the interaction process itself, that is the client, and through the professional's perception of self, as well as by the professional's peer.

Observer Ratings

Rogers (1965, 1975), Truax (1967), Carkhuff (1969), Gazda, Walters, and Childers (1975), and Stetler (1977), among others, have drawn estimates of the professional's ability to offer empathy from observations of professional–client interaction. Carkhuff's *Empathic Understanding in Interpersonal Processes Scale* (1969, Vol. II, pp. 315–317) and the modification of it developed by Gazda and his colleagues (1975), have been used extensively to measure empathy in professional–client interaction (Aspy, 1969; Isquick, 1981; La Monica, Carew, Winder, Haase, and Blanchard, 1976; Layton, 1979; MacKay, Hughes, & Carver, 1981, 1985; Payne, Weiss, & Kapp, 1972; Perry, 1975; Williamson-Kirkland & Williamson-Kirkland,

1980). Mansfield (1973) utilized Truax's Accurate Empathy Scale. Stetler (1977) has developed a content analysis system to categorize sensitive responsiveness of verbal and vocal communicative behaviors of nurses. These behaviors were observed in interviews which were rated most and least empathic, an observational technique to measure empathy indirectly.

An early challenge facing investigators wanting to use an observational system for rating empathic behaviors is to identify those specific behaviors which indicate empathy. How is empathy manifested during professional–client interaction? The answer to this rests on the investigator's operationalization of the concept of empathy. An example follows to illustrate this process.

The construct of empathy utilized by Gazda and others is viewed as having two components. The first is the manifestation of the helping professional's attention to the client's message, both in actions and in words. The professional's response reveals understanding of the content and the feelings of the client's message. It reveals also attitudinal orientations of the professional which may influence the assessment of the client's situation. The second component is seen as the client's perception of the professional's response shown by the client's reply to it, which serves to validate the professional's understanding of the client's message. Thus the use of empathy as observed in dyadic interaction is a two-step process starting from the client's statement—the professional's response followed by the client's reply or further statement.

Inherent in all approaches to the rating of skills of the professional from observed interaction are problems in determining the unit of observation to be rated and inter-judge reliability. Several investigators using observational methods have found that judges do not gain high enough agreement on the assignment of ratings of observed behaviors to achieve reliability of measurement (Layton, 1979; MacKay et al., 1981; Payne et al., 1972; Perry, 1975). On the other hand Williamson-Kirkland and Williamson-Kirkland (1980) reported an interrater reliability of .95 using the Carkhuff-based Human Resources Development Rating Scale.

Three main strategies have been employed to develop adequate interrater reliability. Payne et al. (1972) averaged the ratings of behaviors across two judges assigning the mean value as the score to be used for analysis. Williamson-Kirkland and Williamson-Kirkland (1980, p. 223) employed this tactic also. A second strategy is to gain inter-judge agreement after the training of judges, using responses to a paper and pencil test. The judges subsequently rate the observed behavior of the professional from recorded interactions with a client, either heard directly or from a transcript, or from both. Perry (1975) reported interrater correlations of .82 following training, using the written responses as stimuli, but in the actual performance of judges with observed data interrater reliability dropped to .62. La Monica et al. (1976), using this process, described rater reliability as .83, and Layton (1979) found reliabilities from training ranging from .57 to .99. There is a third strategy which employs an average rating over several observations for a defined segment of the interaction. Perry (1975) increased interrater reliability from .62 to .91 when global ratings of two minute segments of the interaction were made. Payne et al. (1972) also averaged their ratings across six subject responses. Layton (1979) used an average score for a 10 minute segment of interaction which gave a reliability figure of .97.

Although the strategies just cited increase reliability of ratings, serious thought must be given to the effects these strategies have on the data to be analyzed. First of all, a question may be raised about the precision of ratings made by judges when inter-judge reliability was determined by a procedure which was different from that used in the research process itself. If judges cannot agree on the assignment of a rating the training may not be sufficient, or the scale is probably deficient in establishing clear referents for each selected scale category.

Averaged ratings across units in a segment of interaction reduce variability in the data. This decrease in variability usually eliminates measurements at extremes of the scale. In the measurement of empathy using Carkhuff's five-point scale (1969, Vol. II, pp. 315–329) MacKay and colleagues (1985) found the majority of ratings in one particular sample of nurses fell in the level two category, and typically less than ten percent of ratings were found to be higher or lower. Therefore, an average rating representing several observations gives mean scores which produce a homogeneous set of data. Because empathy is very often the independent variable in an investigation, this homogeneity prevents testing of hypotheses about empathy.

Client Perceptions

The most frequently used measure of empathy derived from the client's perspective is the empathy subscale of the Barrett-Lennard

Relationship Inventory (BLRI) (Barrett-Lennard, 1962). The BLRI is an 83-item paper and pencil instrument developed to assess therapeutic change in a therapist–client relationship over time. The fundamental premise underlying the construction of the instrument with its five subscales is the belief that it is the client's experience of the therapist's response which influences therapy (p. 2). Sixteen items constitute the Empathic understanding subscale, and responses are reported on a six-point Likert-type form indicating the degree to which the client perceives each item to be true of the therapist (pp. 34–36). An example of one item (No. 47) is "He appreciates what my experiences feel like to *me*" (p. 35). The BLRI has been used widely to assess the client's perception of the health professional's empathy as determined by the client while receiving professional care (for examples, see Collins, 1972; Forsyth, 1979; Gagan, 1983; Hardin & Halaris, 1983; Kalisch, 1971; Layton, 1979; Stetler, 1977). Other have developed instruments for this purpose as well. For example, see Kalisch (1971) who constructed a predictive accuracy test to infer empathy, modeled after Dymond, which used items from the Minnesota Multiphasic Personality Inventory (p. 205). The Empathy Construct Rating Scale (ECRS) developed by La Monica (1981) is another measure which has been used in investigations of nurse empathy (Bagshaw, 1982/1983; Rogers, 1982; Zimmerman, 1980). La Monica has further developed the ECRS as a new instrument, the La Monica Empathy Profile (1986). This instrument can be used to gain appraisals of usual empathic behaviors of the helping professional by either clients or through the professional's self-appraisal. The appraisal uses a forced-choice response inventory consisting of 30 items. Responses to the items form the basis for the development of a five-dimensional empathy profile indicative of the professional's usual repertoire in demonstrating empathic behavior.

Gagan (1983) summarized the principal difficulties found in nursing studies using reports of patient perceptions: (a) patients perceive nurses as empathic whether they are or not, evidenced by high correlations with patient satisfaction and low correlations with empathy training; (b) the BLRI assumes the professional–client relationship to be sustained over time, whereas in nursing, especially in hospital nursing, relationships are often of short duration so that the patient does not know the nurse well enough to respond to the questions asked on the BLRI; and (c) patients are a captive group and may be deterred from offering candid responses through concerns for their subsequent care. Added to these difficulties is the fact that retrospective data are subject to all the distortions of recall which plague any history-taking assessment situation.

Professionals' Self-rating

Self-rating scales frequently have been used to measure the empathy of professional care givers (Brunt, 1985; Dagenais & Meleis, 1982; D'Augelli, 1973; Diseker & Michielutte, 1981; Elizur & Rosenheim, 1982; Forsyth, 1979; Hogan, 1969; Kalisch, 1971; Kirk, 1978/1979; Kunst-Wilson, Carpenter, Poser, Venohr, & Kushner, 1981; La Monica, 1981; Streit-Forest, 1982). Hogan's Empathy Scale (1969) is discussed as an illustration. It is a self-report scale which has been employed in several studies, for example by Brunt (1985), Diseker and Michielutte (1981), and Forsyth (1979). The scale consists of 64 statements which respondents claim to be true or false relative to their self-appraisals. Hogan described a number of steps in evaluating the scale in terms of validity and reliability. Subsequent utilization by others gives further evidence of its value in the investigation of empathy.

The major criticism of self-report scales is that most depend on an intellectual self-appraisal of ability which may not be borne out behaviorally. To substantiate this criticism, both D'Augelli (1973, p. 179) and Kunst-Wilson et al. (1981, p. 288) can be cited. They found no agreement between self-reports of empathic ability and observer ratings of actual ability. Some self-report scales include a cognitive component (for example see Layton, 1979) and this raises further questions regarding the capability of a scale which measures one characteristic to predict behaviors which may emanate from other characteristics. Knowledge is in general an imperfect predictor of performance because other factors, such as self-image, motivation, values, and environmental conditions intervene to modify outcome. For a discussion of the inability of knowledge to predict medical compliance, see Haynes (1976) who has written extensively about compliance with medical regimens.

Peer Ratings

The professional's ability to offer empathy, as perceived by peers or by supervisory personnel, has been the basis of the measurement of empathy in some studies. La Monica (1981) examined ratings of empathy by the nurse's peers, as well as by the client and self-ratings by the nurse, using the Empathy Construct Rating Scale (ECRS) she developed. The ECRS is an evaluation of the feelings or actions the professional has toward another person, using a Likert-type paper and pencil response format over 100 items (p. 390). Correlations between peer and self ratings, and self with client ratings, were low but significant.

D'Augelli (1973) also has studied empathy as evaluated by peers, as well as by trained observers and the professional's view of self-performance. He modified the Group Assessment of Interpersonal Trait (GAIT) instrument developed by Goodman, which uses inter-personal behavior in a small group as the basis for study. Findings revealed a low but significant agreement between observer and peer ratings of empathy, but peer–self and observer–self ratings were not significantly related.

A study by Kirk (1978/1979) of psychiatric nurses before and after an empathy training program showed supervisor's ratings of the nurses to be inconsistent with nurses' self-ratings and ratings by clients. Several scales were used in these assessments.

These studies show peer (or supervisors') ratings to be poorly correlated with observer and self-ratings, which may be one reason why there appear to be few studies reported which depend on peer ratings alone.

Tests Inferring Ability to Offer Empathy

Tests have been developed to infer the ability of the professional to offer empathy to a client. Notable among these are Carkhuff's Indices of Communication and Discrimination (1969) and Truax's Accurate Empathy Scale (1967). Both have been used extensively by others. For an example of the use of Carkhuff's Scale, see Farrell, Haley, and Magnasco (1977), Isquick (1981); La Monica (1981), La Monica, et al., (1976), Williamson-Kirkland and Williamson-Kirkland (1980), and Valle (1981). Kalisch (1971) and Natale (1972) report studies using Truax's Scale. These paper and pencil tests require the respondent to generate responses to client statements which are rated on the selected scale by judges who have been trained previously in the use of the scale and were found to give reliable ratings. Reliability is typically established through interrater agreement in excess of .80.

The use of paper and pencil tests offers distinct advantages in ease of gaining data at reasonable cost as well as reliability of measurements. However, there are some concerns. The client situation is simulated either by acting it out in a laboratory situation or depicting it in a written description. The professional verbalizes or writes responses to client statements which are standard stimuli from which inferences regarding ability to offer empathy are made. There is, therefore, the implicit inference that the professional's ability will transfer to the practice setting. Kurtz and Grummon (1972) discuss this factor. Several investigators show that this transfer of ability is not assured (for discussion of this see Bath & Calhoun, 1977; Farrell, et al., 1977). Moreover, scale validity may be another concern. Rappaport and Chinsky claim that Truax's Accurate Empathy Scale lacks discriminant validity (1972, p. 400), because therapist warmth and genuineness ratings correlated equally as well with a 7-point semantic differential dimension of understanding/not understanding as did the empathy ratings (pp. 400–401). This criticism, however, was based on the use of ratings of segments of audiotaped therapist vocalizations rather than judgments of written responses to a standardized client statement, although this distinction is probably not important.

EMPATHY MEASURED
AS A PERSONALITY ATTRIBUTE

Conceptually distinct from the behaviorists are those who view empathy as emanating from the individual's personality. Hogan (1975) discusses empathy in terms of its role in interpersonal conduct and in moral development. He developed his scale (1969) to distinguish the person who is socially perceptive, aware of impressions made on others, from the one who relates to everyone in the same way, in socially desirable or conventional terms (1975, p. 15). Hogan's scale, discussed earlier as a means of gaining the professional's self-appraisal of ability, has had wide use from investigators using a personality perspective of empathy. See, for example, Brunt (1985), Diseker and Michielutte (1981), Forsyth (1979), and Streit-Forest (1982). Hogan's Scale is one of the better known measures of empathy from a personality perspective. However, psychologists differ widely in their conceptual approaches to personality.

One of the interesting developments in the work of psychologists in the study of empathy is the view that empathy can be seen to stem from external sources, that is, situational or interpersonal contexts, termed state empathy or phenotypic empathy, as well as from internal sources, that is, the more stable personality attributes, termed trait or genotypic empathy (Hogan, 1975, p. 17). The trait empathy is subject to measurement by the Hogan Scale, whereas the state empathy is amenable to a behavioral measure using an observer perspective. Steibe, Boulet, and Lee (1979) also distinguish trait empathy from state empathy. They used the BLRI to estimate empathic functioning viewed as state empathy, and the empathy/egocentrism scale (P) of the Comrey Personality Scales to measure trait empathy. They say that individuals who score high on the P Scale rate themselves as sympathetic, helpful, generous, unselfish, and interested in other people.

Measurement of empathy as a personality factor is not always measured in a direct way. Several psychologists have used experimental situations in the study of empathy (for example, Batson, Coke, & Pych, 1983; Batson, O'Quin, Fultz, Vanderplas, & Isen, 1983; Coke, Batson, & McDavis, 1978; Rothenberg, 1984/1985; Toi, & Batson, 1982). Empathy as the maneuver is manipulated in the experiment with various outcomes examined, helping behavior being one outcome of central interest to several investigators. Batson and his colleagues have studied dispositional empathy and altruism in this way, designing empathy-inducing situations to force subject participants to act in a manner to reveal their altruistic motivations.

EMPATHY MEASURED
AS EXPERIENCED EMOTION

Some psychologists have conceptualized empathy as the experienced emotions of others. Stotland, Mathews, Sherman, Hansson, and Richardson (1978) note that when the observer's responses to someone watched have the same valence or emotional direction, the response is described as simple empathy (p. 12). Their Fantasy–Empathy (F–E) Scale used to measure simple empathy is a self-reported paper and pencil test which indicates the direction of an emotional response to test situations. The F–E Scale is based on three items with a reported test—retest reliability of 0.83 (p. 42).

Mehrabian and Epstein (1972) developed a questionnaire to measure empathic tendency and this scale has been used frequently by others (for example Elizur & Rosenheim, 1982; Watson, Hood, Morris, & Hall, 1984; Williams, 1982). The 33-item scale employs an 8-point response format to reveal emotional empathy. In illustration, Item 1 states "It makes me sad to see a lonely stranger in a group" (Mehrabian & Ebstein, p. 528). The split-half reliability was reported to be .84 (p. 527), and the scale was deemed highly reliable (p. 540) and valid in quite distinct settings (p. 542).

Emotional empathy, however, is not always viewed as conceptually clear, and the measurement processes which stem from the concept can offer variable interpretations. Cognitive empathy is thought by some psychologists to be distinct from empathy as an emotion. Shantz (1975) discusses understanding and feeling in respect to empathy, noting that measures to tap these constructs must be different. Iannotti (1975) also notes that in some experiments reported in the literature subjects can interpret variously the enacted scenarios, ignoring emotional cues to give a strictly cognitive response to the experimental situation (p. 23).

SUMMARY

Review of the research literature on empathy shows several different perspectives of the construct of empathy to have influenced the development of its measurement. The major means of measurement are: (a) observer ratings, (b) client perceptions, (c) professionals' self-ratings, (d) peer ratings, (e) tests inferring ability to offer empathy, (f) personality measures, (g) experimental manipulation of enacted empathy to study the observer's response, and (h) tests to assess the experienced emotion of the observer in a situation created to invoke empathy. The advantages and disadvantages of these various approaches were discussed in relation to a designated measurement need.

Accountability in professional practice requires the assessment of clinical ability. Competence in clinical practice is dependent on the ability of the professional to interact therapeutically with the client. The need to assess communication skills is essential to identify competence, and the measurement of empathy is of central concern.

Lack of consensus on the means of measuring empathy has

blocked the progress of research into the effects of the professional's use of empathy in professional–client interaction on the subsequent wellbeing of the client. Until this obstacle is surmounted research in this area of professional practice will lag.

REFERENCES

Aspy, D. N. (1969). The effect of teacher-offered conditions of empathy, positive regard, and congruence upon student achievement. *Florida Journal of Educational Research, 11,* 39–48.

Bagshaw, M. Y. (1982/1983). Geriatric nurses' attitudes, empathy, and ideologic orientation. (From *Dissertation Abstracts International,* 1983, *43,* Abstract No. 2854B.)

Barrett-Lennard, G. T. (1962). Dimensions of therapist response as causal factors in therapeutic change. *Psychological Monographs, 76* (43, Whole No. 562).

Bath, K. E., & Calhoun, R. O. (1977). The effects of professional counselor training on empathy: Continued cause for concern. *Counselor Education and Supervision, 17,* 98–106.

Batson, C. D., Coke, J. S., & Pych, V. (1983). Limits on the two-stage model of empathic mediation of helping: A reply to Archer, Diaz-Loving, Gollwitzer, Davis and Foushee. *Journal of Personality and Social Psychology, 45,* 895–898.

Batson C. D., O'Quin, K., Fultz, J., & Vanderplas, M. (1983). Influence of self-reported distress and empathy on egoistic versus altruistic motivation to help. *Journal of Personality and Social Psychology, 45,* 706–718.

Brunt, J. H. (1985). An exploration of the relationship between nurses' empathy and technology. *Nursing Administration Quarterly, 9*(4), 69–78.

Carkhuff, R. R. (1969). *Helping and human relations: A primer for lay and professional helpers* (Vols. I & II). New York: Holt Rinehart & Winston.

Coke, J. S., Batson, C. D., & McDavis, K. (1978). Empathic mediation of helping: A two-stage model. *Journal of Personality and Social Psychology, 36,* 752–766.

Collins, D. L. (1972). *Empathic ability and dogmatism in nursing students.* Unpublished doctoral dissertation, Teachers College, Columbia University, New York.

Dagenais, R., & Meleis, A. I. (1982). Professionalism, work ethic, and empathy in nursing: The nurse self-description form. *Western Journal of Nursing Research, 4,* 407–422.

D'Augelli, A. R. (1973). The assessment of interpersonal skills: A comparison of observer, peer, and self ratings. *Journal of Community Psychology 1,* 177–179.

Diseker, R. A., & Michielutte, R. (1981). An analysis of empathy in medical students before and following clinical experience. *Journal of Medical Education*, 56, 1004–1010.

Elizur, A., & Rosenheim, E. (1982). Empathy and attitudes among medical students: The effects of group experience. *Journal of Medical Education*, 57, 675–683.

Farrell, M., Haley, M., & Magnasco, J. (1977). Teaching interpersonal skills. *Nursing Outlook*, 25, 322–325.

Forsyth, G. L. (1979). Exploration of empathy in nurse–client interaction. *Advances in Nursing Science*, 1(2), 53–61.

Gagan, J. M. (1983). Methodological notes on empathy. *Advances in Nursing Science*, 5(2), 65–72.

Gazda, G. M., Walters, R. P., & Childers, W. C. (1975). *Human relations development*. Boston: Allyn & Bacon.

Hardin, S. B., & Halaris, A. L. (1983). Nonverbal communication of patients and high and low empathy nurses. *Journal of Psychosocial Nursing and Mental Health Services*, 21(1), 14–20.

Haynes, R. B. (1976). Strategies for improving compliance: Methodological analysis and review. In D. L. Sackett & R. B. Haynes (Eds.), *Compliance and therapeutic regimens*. (pp. 121–143). Baltimore: Johns Hopkins University Press.

Hogan, R. (1969). Development of an empathic scale. *Journal of Consulting and Clinical Psychology*, 33, 307–316.

Hogan, R. (1975). Empathy: A conceptual and psychometric analysis. *The Counseling Psychologist*, 5(2), 14–18.

Iannotti, R. J. (1975). The nature and measurement of empathy in children. *The Counseling Psychologist*, 5(2), 21–25.

Isquick, M. F. (1981). Training older people in empathy: Effects on empathy, attitudes, and self-exploration. *International Journal of Aging and Human Development*, 13(1), 1–14.

Kalisch, B. J. (1971). An experiment in the development of empathy in nursing students. *Nursing Research*, 20, 202–211.

Kirk, W. G. (1978/1979). The effect of interpersonal process recall method training and interpersonal communication training on the empathic behavior of psychiatric nursing personnel. (From *Dissertation Abstracts International*, 1979, 39, Abstract No. 3522B).

Kunst-Wilson, W., Carpenter, L., Poser, A., Venohr, I., & Kushner, K. (1981). Empathic perceptions of nursing students: Self-reported and actual ability. *Research in Nursing and Health*, 4, 283–293.

Kurtz, R. R., & Grummon, D. L. (1972). Different approaches to the measurement of therapist empathy and their relationship to therapy outcomes. *Journal of Consulting and Clinical Psychology*, 39, 106–115.

La Monica, E. L. (1981). Construct validity of an empathic instrument. *Research in Nursing and Health*, 4, 389–400.

La Monica, E. L., Carew, D. K., Winder, A. E., Haase, A. M. B., &

Blanchard, K. H. (1976). Empathy training as the major thrust of a staff development program. *Nursing Research, 25,* 447–451.

La Monica, E. L. (1986). *La Monica Empathy Profile.* Tuxedo, NY: XICOM.

Layton, J. M. (1979). The use of modeling to teach empathy to nursing students. *Research in Nursing and Health, 2,* 163–176.

MacKay, R. C., Hughes, J., & Carver, E. J. (1981). *Nurse–patient communication in a burn unit.* Unpublished report, Dalhousie University, Halifax.

MacKay, R. C., Hughes, J., & Carver, E. J. (1985). The nurse's use of empathy as it affects the stress and self-disclosures of patients with burns or other accidental wounds, a pilot study. *The Bulletin and Clinical Review of Burn Injuries, 2,*(1), 43–44.

Mansfield, E. (1973). Empathy: Concept and identified psychiatric nursing behavior. *Nursing Research, 22,* 525–530.

Mehrabian, A., & Epstein, N. (1972). A measure of emotional empathy. *Journal of Personality, 40,* 525–543.

Natale, S. (1972). *An experiment in empathy.* Windsor, Berks: National Foundation for Educational Research in England and Wales.

Payne, P. A., Weiss, S. D., & Kapp, R. A. (1972). Didactic, experiential, and modeling factors in the learning of empathy. *Journal of Counseling Psychology, 19,* 425–429.

Perry, M. A. (1975). Modeling and instructions in training for counselor empathy. *Journal of Counseling Psychology, 22,* 173–179.

Rappaport, J., & Chinsky, J. M. (1972). Accurate empathy: Confusion of a construct. *Psychological Bulletin, 77,* 400–404.

Rogers, C. R. (1965). *Client-centered therapy.* Boston: Houghton Mifflin.

Rogers, C. R. (1975). Empathic: An unappreciated way of being. *The Counseling Psychologist, 5*(2), 2–10.

Rogers, I. A. (1982). Effects of undergraduate nursing education on empathy. (From *Dissertation Abstracts International,* 1982, *43,* Abstract No. 1436B).

Rothenberg, S. H. (1984/1985). Empathy and sacrifice as factors in altruistic helping of sixth-grade girls. (From *Dissertation Abstracts International,* 1985, *45,* Abstract No. 3657B.)

Shantz, C. U. (1975). Empathy in relation to social cognitive development. *The Counseling Psychologist, 5*(2), 18–21.

Steibe, S. C., Boutlet, D. B., & Lee, D. C. (1979). Trainee trait empathy, age, trainer functioning, client age and training time as discriminators of successful empathy training. *Canadian Counsellor, 14*(1), 41–46.

Stetler, C. B. (1977). Relationship of perceived empathy to nurses' communication. *Nursing Research, 26,* 432–438.

Stotland, E., Mathews, K. E., Jr., Sherman, S. E., Hansson, R. O., & Richardson, B. Z. (1978). *Empathy, fantasy and helping.* Beverly Hills: Sage.

Streit-Forest U. (1982). Differences in empathy: A preliminary analysis.

    Journal of Medical Education, 57(1), 65–67.
Toi, M., & Batson, C. D. (1982). More evidence that empathy is a source
    of altuistic motivation. *Journal of Personality and Social Psychology,*
    43, 281–292.
Truax, C. (1967). A scale for rating of accurate empathy. In C. R. Rogers,
    E. Gendlin, D. Kiesler, & C. B. Truax (Eds.), *The therapeutic relationship*
    and its impact: A study of psychotherapy with schizophrenics. Madison:
    University of Wisconsin Press.
Valle, S. K. (1981). Interpersonal functioning of alcoholism counselors and
    treatment outcome. *Journal of Studies on Alcohol, 42,* 783–790.
Watson, P. J., Hood, R. W., Morris, R. J., & Hall, J. R. (1984). Empathy,
    religious orientation, and social desirability. *The Journal of Psychology*
    117, 211–216.
Williams, C. L. (1979). Empathic communication and its effect on client
    outcome. *Issues in Mental Health Nursing, 2*(1), 15–26.
Williamson-Kirkland, T. E., & Williamson-Kirkland, R. H. (1980). Teaching
    communication skills in rehabilitation medicine. *Archives of Physical*
    Medicine and Rehabilitation, 61, 221–224.
Zimmerman, B. M. (1980). Teaching empathy to baccalaureate nursing
    students. (From *Dissertation Abstracts International,* 1980, *41,* Abstract
    No. 1314B.)

AUTHORS' NOTE

This chapter draws on a paper given at the ninth National Conference,
Nursing Research: A Base for Practice, October 12–14, 1983, Montreal, Canada, and subsequently published in the *Special Supplement of Nursing Pa-*
pers, 1984, 160–169. Used with permission of *Nursing Papers.*

Part III

Empathy in Health Care Practice: An Examination of Nurse–Patient Interaction in a Hospital Acute Care Setting

The focus of Part Three is on empathy as it is relevant to health care practice, and more specifically, nursing in a hospital acute care setting. This section describes the Empathy Study Program, a program of research in nursing practice extending over several years in a Burn Unit and the associated plastic surgery nursing unit.

Chapter 8 outlines the early studies leading to the need to develop an empathy training program for nurses in the Burn Unit. The training program and its evaluation are described.

Chapters 9 and 10 focus on the subsequent study of empathy in nurse–patient interaction as it affects patient care outcomes. Chapter 9 discusses the assessment of the impact of nurse empathy on patient self-disclosures through a microanalysis of the interaction. In Chapter 10 attention is given to the qual-

itative evaluation of the same dialogue to reveal characteristics of conversation which are reflective of higher levels of empathy as distinct from lower levels.

8

Learning to Use Empathy

Jean R. Hughes
E. Joyce Carver
Ruth C. MacKay

Intuitive abilities will not enable most people to give sustained high level empathic responses. The literature reports many helping professionals are unable to demonstrate empathy at a facilitative level (Carkhuff, 1969a; Gagan, 1983; Kalisch, 1971; La Moncia, Carew, Winder, Haase, & Blanchard, 1976; Layton, 1979; Payne, Weiss, & Kapp, 1972; Peitchinis, 1972, 1976; Williamson-Kirkland & Williamson-Kirkland, 1980). Although not all studies concur with these results (La Monica & Karshmer, 1978; Rogers, 1986), the conflict may be due more to conceptual difficulties and the use of different measures of empathy than to actual performance. How can professionals acquire this communication ability? A specific approach for teaching the skill of empathy to nurses is described in this chapter, including the structural components of a particular training program and an analysis of the changes observed in the learners as the program progressed.

The training program was developed in response to the need to raise the level of empathic functioning of nurses giving direct patient care. Ultimately we wished to examine the effects of high and low empathy on patient care outcomes. Training in the use of empathy by practicing professionals is an expensive process, and unless justified in terms of the ensuing quality of patient care, may not receive the attention it merits. A program of research was developed to examine these merits in a hospital acute care setting, namely a combined burn and plastic surgery nursing unit.

THE EMPATHY RESEARCH PROGRAM

Nurses working in this unit are consistently confronted by challenging working conditions. Not only must they bear considerable physical strain while caring for such patients, by reason of the very warm room temperature, the wearing of extra clothing for isolation precautions, and the long standing required to carry out treatment procedures, but often the environment is emotionally charged as well.

Patients with severe trauma are very sick, sometimes coping with chemical imbalances which affect their behaviors, and very often experiencing severe pain. In addition, there may be worry about survival, the management of the recovery process, loneliness caused by their isolation from others, and concern about the future in terms of how different they may be and how this will affect their lives, their work, and their families. Overwhelming anger and feelings of helplessness are not uncommon. Interventions need the meticulous attention of the nurse, and inevitably the treatments inflict increased pain on patients already stressed and suffering. The burden on the nurse is great, yet more than ever the need to communicate effectively exists. Nurses in the Burn Unit of the Victoria General Hospital in Halifax, Canada voiced concern about the problems they experienced in giving emotional care to the severely burned.

PRELIMINARY STUDY

Observations over a 24-hour period confirmed the nurses' impressions. A preliminary study[1] was mounted which described how nurses gave emotional care to burned patients under the adverse conditions previously identified. Recorded nurse responses in 17

[1]The investigators, R. C. MacKay and R. E. Dennison, acknowledge the assistance of M. Linehan and the Victoria General Hospital, Halifax, Nova Scotia, in the collection of data from some observed interactions.

nurse–patient interactions were classified into five categories: judgments, explanations, questions, sympathy, and empathy.

Judgments and sympathy each occurred 9 percent of the time. Explanations occurred 39 percent, questions were raised 19 percent, and empathy was demonstrated 24 percent of the time. However, when empathy was considered qualitatively, there were no instances when it was given at a facilitative level using Carkhuff's Scale of Empathic Understanding in Interpersonal Processes (1969b, pp. 315–317). That is, the nurse did not show understanding of the patient through verbal recognition of both content and affective dimensions of the patient's message. The distribution found here is quite similar to what has been reported previously by Graffam (1970).

It is important to note that nurses recognized the need to offer empathy about one-quarter of the time. The cue the patient gave as one who suffered in some manner and who was in need of understanding was recognized. The fact that nurses did not act on this cue to offer facilitative communication revealed the need for training in empathy skills, necessary for the observation of the effects of empathy on patient care outcomes.

THE NEED FOR EMPATHY TRAINING

The professional should not leave interpersonal skills to chance. Much of a profession's image is portrayed through verbal presentation, the medium through which expectations are established and met in any relationship (Lambert, 1982). Empathy is one of the principal dimensions employed by helping professionals in communicating with clients (Aiken & Aiken, 1973; Carkhuff, 1969a; Dagenais & Meleis, 1982; Farrell, Haley, & Magnasco, 1977; Gagan, 1983; Gazda, Walters, & Childers, 1975; Gazda, Childers, & Walters, 1982; Kalisch, 1971; La Monica, 1981; La Monica et al., 1976; Layton, 1979; Peitchinis, 1972; Perry, 1975; Stetler, 1977; Williamson-Kirkland & Williamson-Kirkland, 1980). It is considered the most important dimension in the interaction process influencing the emotional care nurses are able to offer patients (Layton, 1978, pp. 5–6, 17), and believed to affect treatment outcomes (for example Lambert, 1982).

Carkhuff (1969a) states that the professional's skill in communicating empathy can actually be harmful if it is not at a basic facilitative level. Rogers' (1986) review of the literature provides ample evidence that the skill of empathy can be learned. It was believed that a training program designed to assist the nurses in the Burn and Plastic Surgery nursing unit regarding the development of empathy, could increase the overall effectiveness of their interactions with others.

THE EMPATHY SKILL TRAINING PROGRAM

The program was created to promote the skills of identification and verbal verification of content and affective components of client messages. The program was offered twice, the first time in 12 sessions and the second for 16 sessions. The program design was similar for both groups of learners; however, the second group allowed for planned absenteeism. Participants received 20–25 hours of planned instruction, experiential learning, modeling, and feedback.

The program was designed to allow participants an opportunity to devote their full attention to the learning process. Therefore, weekly two-hour sessions were held in the university nearby to avoid competition from the demands of the work setting. The instructor was skilled in teaching interpersonal skills and chose a human relations training approach adapted for the program. The manual by Gazda et al. (1975) was used as a supplementary text.

Subjects

Eleven registered nurses volunteered to participate in the demonstration program. All were female and under 44 years of age. Nine had diploma preparation while two had a baccalaureate degree in nursing.

Structural Components

The operational definition of empathy chosen for the training program was that of La Monica (1981).

> Empathy signifies a central focus and feeling *with* and *in* the client's world. It involves accurate perception of the client's world by the helper, communication of this understanding to the client, and the client's perception of the helper's understanding (p. 398).

The literature describes a number of interpersonal skill development programs conducted with nurses in which empathy is a dominant focus (Anderson & Gerrard, 1984; Farrell, Haley, & Magnasco, 1977; Kalisch, 1971; La Monica, 1983; La Monica, Madea & Oberst, 1987; Steibe, Boulet & Lee, 1979; Williamson-Kirkland & Williamson-Kirkland, 1980). These range in length from six to 45 hours and include the common features of didactic instruction, experiential learning, modeling behavior, rehearsal, and feedback. Therefore, our empathy training program was similar.

Content incorporated a general overview of the helping relationship theory, communication theory, the helping relationship model described by Gazda and colleagues (1975), perception and its communication to others, specific dimensions of empathy as a learned skill and personality attribute, and role responsibilities of the nurse in relation to empathy. A group approach was chosen as it provided the opportunity to observe the behavior of others, share in feedback given to others, practice skills in a mutually supportive atmosphere, and get the maximum benefits from a minimum expenditure of time and energy (Carkhuff, 1969b, p. 181).

Flexible design was integrated to respond to participant concerns regarding the intellectual and emotional demands of the program. The focus moved from the discussion of factual content to process-oriented sessions involving problem-solving of actual client situations introduced by participants. These situations were representative of central issues facing clinical nurses daily.

The first two-hour session included an orientation to the program, signing the individual consent forms, and a pretest of the initial abilities of nurses to use empathy in a laboratory situation. Subsequent training sessions followed at weekly intervals. The final session provided opportunity for the post-training evaluation of the participants and the program itself.

Sessions were rigorous, and a 15-minute debriefing period, conducted by a person other than the instructor, was included at the end of each session. This provided a planned transition between the program and the workplace. Empathy training involves the need for behavior changes which affect the learner's self-image, self-esteem, and perception of professional competence. Recognizing the need for behavior changes in nurses who are otherwise considered to be highly skilled can be expected to evoke strong reactions. Opportunity to explore these responses with someone outside of the training session, and yet confidential to the group, was considered a very important safeguard in the management of the total educational program. The investigator responsible for the debriefing anticipated emotional reactions and role-modeled empathic responses to help the nurses explore their experiences.

The program progressed in its intensity in a manner similar to that of an effective helping relationship, that is, from the less threatening to the more sensitive subject matter. The first few sessions were quite structured and incorporated teacher-designed paper and pencil exercises, similar to those suggested by Gazda and colleagues (1975), requiring participants to write empathic responses to videotaped client statements. This provided tangible feedback regarding cues missed or avoided. Gradually the same objective was achieved through role playing with partners and writing exercises were eliminated. The activity permitted an experience in both giving and receiving assistance and, in most cases, a deeper appreciation of the client role as well. A similar activity is described by La Monica (1983) in her use of the process of imagery. She believes the more "nurses have experienced another's world, the greater likelihood that caring will be communicated" (p. 20).

Finally, the role-playing exercises were videotaped and reviewed in group discussions, to improve the quality and quantity of feedback available to participants about their performance. Videotaping is a painfully uncensored exposure of one's skills; however, it does provide comprehensive feedback in a way that is not possible through memory recall. Participants soon recognized the difficulty involved in both listening and making oneself understood. As well they realized how misunderstandings could result from a series of small but inaccurate assumptions resulting from failure to validate client messages.

Issues became the focus in later sessions where learners addressed matters of emotional and ethical concern. Participants examined troublesome situations brought from the work place and the group collaborated on problem-solving strategies. Attention was given to enhancing the nurses' understanding of client behavior in traumatic circumstances (in this case those associated with burns) and how it in turn affects the interaction patterns of the professionals involved. It was recognized that burns are among the most devastating of all injuries, as individuals are left with permanent reminders of the impact to their physical and emotional selves (Black, 1986). Consequently, it was crucial that the participants had insight concerning the complexities of the situations in which they were expected to interact effectively.

How Learning Evolved

From anxiety and skepticism to commitment

During the early sessions learners were visibly anxious about the program activities. They were skeptical of the instructor's credibility and of the relevance and impact that empathy could have on their relationships with clients. Such reactions are typical of learners according to Morton and Kurtz (1982), as students actively resist any activity which might threaten their identity. Participants were asked to examine their empathy skills in detail. As this often moved to a more comprehensive exploration of all communication skills, discomfort was expected and addressed openly by the instructor.

It became clear that attention had to be placed on the process of change occurring in the learners as they acquired new skills. Duldt (1981, 1982) notes the importance of control in the alleviation of anxiety in nurses. The structure of the early sessions provided direction and purpose and consequently served as a form of security for the participants. In later sessions, when nurses were asked to role-play, they were encouraged to assume responsibility for situation development in an effort to affirm their input and ultimate command of their own learning. Although supplementary readings were identified throughout the program as another avenue for self-directed learning, participants generally took advantage of these resources only after committing themselves to the significance of empathy in their interactions with others. This tended to occur during later sessions.

The program became viable when participants were willing to risk themselves. "The degree of involvement in a relationship refers not only to the amount of interaction between participants, but also to the importance each attaches to this interaction" (Duldt, Giffin, & Patton, 1984, p. 123). The degree of importance became obvious as the nurses started identifying their own learning needs and the activities became more learner-directed. The participants were beginning to develop a sense of ownership about the program and grant it credibility. They were willing to test the application of empathy on a limited basis in their work setting, to evaluate its significance in the "real world." This indicated the nurses' willingness to expose awkward attempts with a new skill in front of peers. The commitment to the program began to solidify. The nurse-initiated role-playing interactions on videotape grew longer and more complex, and the feedback regarding empathy skill performance evolved in terms of its specificity and comprehensiveness. Discussions centered on the importance of receiving constructive feedback from peers and on the awareness of a sense of fellowship with colleagues.

From facts to issues

From the hypothetical to reality

As issues became the focus of the later sessions, participants felt more comfortable in exposing their feelings of inadequacy in addressing complex matters such as anger, silence, and helplessness. In order to achieve a satisfying resolution of these dilemmas it was crucial to understand the circumstances inherent in the situation from the perspective of both the patient and the nurse. For example, in many instances the nurse was seen to represent pain to clients. Her presence would generate their loud outbursts of angry protest in comments such as, "Not you again! With you around, seems no one can get any rest."

"At times, nursing care inevitably involves discomfort for the client. . . . [and] anger generally occurs in response to the frustration and anxiety that result when an individual is unable to fulfill a need or reach a goal" (Sundeen, Stuart, Rankin, & Cohen, 1985, p. 187). The nurse's reaction in this circumstance often resulted in her becoming a victim and seeking refuge in defensive behavior. Rather than acknowledging the anger through empathy, the nurse might make comments which either rationalized her interventions such as, "You really need all of this treatment to get better", or reprimanded the client, "If you didn't complain so much I think you would find that the treatment wouldn't be so bad!" Duldt and her colleagues (Duldt, 1984, p. 219) suggest that such behavior occurs when individuals perceive other's communication as an attempt to control. The interchanges in this type of encounter often became cyclical and obviously had little therapeutic value.

Another situation nurses often chose to address in the laboratory program was that of patient-expressed helplessness. The endless hours of painful treatment they endured and the distortion of the body image their wounds created became overwhelming for clients. Eventually even the most stoic individuals succumbed to feelings of desperation. It is understandable how those emotions transferred to the nurses who, despite their best efforts, could not magically eliminate the devastating effects of such trauma. Control is very important in alleviating a sense of helplessness (Duldt, 1982). However, rather than acknowledging this feeling through empathy, the nurse often responded with actions that made the client dependent through comments such as, " Don't worry. Everything is going to be all right." The false reassurance reflected the nurse's own sense of powerlessness and served to undermine the legitimacy of the client's feelings. This tended to result in client outrage, increased dependency, or withdrawal.

Participants found that the re-creation of actual situations reflecting issues experienced in the workplace facilitated the application of empathy theory. Although the role playing focused mainly on the skill of empathy, general consultation regarding the theory of behavior was clearly required. It enabled learners to develop their analytical skills as they gained better understanding of the situational dynamics. These sessions provided an opportunity for the individual nurse to realize that her sources of difficulty had many similarities to those of her peers. Unfortunately, most participants had not felt comfortable disclosing their concerns to peers in the past nor had they been encouraged to do so. These nurses seemed to view the act of consultation as a sign of personal failure and weak professional practice.

As the program progressed, the learners made a request to examine problematic colleagial relationships. Many nurses felt immobilized by stressful confrontations as they believed that demonstrating low-risk behavior with clients and maintaining a non-controversial position on the health team would be less intimidating. These behaviors reinforced the status quo and met expectations of the surrounding environment (Kelly, 1981; Omery, 1983). Unfortunately, this low risk behavior was no match for encounters with short-tempered colleagues and caused the nurses to feel powerless. They recognized the potential for negative consequences on vulnerable client interactions if they failed to acknowledge their concerns regarding peer interactions. Participants began to observe and evaluate the interaction patterns of colleagues on the health team. They developed heightened sensitivity to the appropriate use of empathy for creating effective encounters.

RESULTS OF THE TRAINING PROGRAM

The effectiveness of the training program in assisting nurses to use empathy was evaluated in terms of the changes in ratings of empathy calculated before and after the training program. An adaptation of Carkhuff's Empathetic Understanding in Interpersonal Processes Scale (1969b, pp. 315–317) modified by Gazda and his colleagues (1975) was used for this purpose.

Measurements were made by judges using pre- and post-tests of learner–client recorded interaction. The pre- and post-testing was done in a laboratory setting. Participants viewed simulated male client situations recorded on videotape. They were asked to provide written responses to four statements which could be expected to require empathy from the nurse. Following the written part, learners interacted in person with a female simulated client and were videotaped while making spoken responses to four standard statements. The test was the same for both pre- and post-measurements of empathy. It is recognized that factors could have influenced the subjects' abilities, either through a self-conscious attitude to the observational process, thus lowering demonstrated skill level, or by increasing the level through unusual attention to skills not exercised in an ordinary, non-laboratory, client situation. No attempt was made to influence these potential reactions.

Interrater reliability was developed through nine hours of practice in rating the professional's responses in their interactions with clients. A reliability of .92 was demonstrated on written responses and 1.0 on spoken responses using Scott's coefficient of agreement, correlating the judge's and trainer's independent ratings. Thereafter the one judge made all ratings.

Empathy ratings before the training program and at its conclusion yielded four ratings for each trainee on both written and spoken responses pre- and post-training. A score derived from these eight responses provided data for the pre- and post-tests. The mean rating on written responses at the pretest was 2.075 and on the spoken test it was 2.05. Some nurses responded initially at a level one, which shows that they were unable to avoid periodic hurtful or psychologically damaging types of reactions. This is consistent with other noted observations reported in the literature with other nurses and helping professionals (Carkhuff, 1969a, pp. 145-155; La Monica et al., 1976; Layton, 1979).

The post-training ratings showed increased ability to use empathy. All subjects increased their abilities on all sections of both the written and spoken tests. The mean rating on the written post-test was 2.975 and on the spoken test it was 2.875. Subjected to statistical analysis using the Wilcoxon matched pairs signed ranks test the probability of such changes occurring by chance was less than .005. The fact that changes were consistent throughout the group adds clinical significance to this finding. All nurses were able to offer empathic responses at a helpful level to the simulated patient. A further test of retention was conducted seven months following the program and demonstrated no significant decline in empathy skill.

CONCLUSION

Clearly the participants in the Empathy Training Program demonstrated their skill in applying empathy effectively in the laboratory setting. However such a program must attend to much more than skill acquisition. The application of empathy is dependent on a number of factors. Those factors influencing empathy and its transfer to practice are delineated further in Chapters 6 and 12. A discussion of the effects of empathy on client well-being is contained in the next chapter.

REFERENCES

Aiken, L., & Aiken, J. L. (1973). A systematic approach to the evaluation of interpersonal relationships. *American Journal of Nursing, 73*, 863–867.

Anderson, H., & Gerrard, B. (1984). A comprehensive interpersonal skills program for nurses. *Journal of Nursing Education, 23*(8), 353–355.

Black, J. (1986). Burns. In C. R. Kneisl, & S. W. Ames (Eds.), *Adult health nursing: A biopychosocial approach* (pp. 439–475). Menlo Park, CA: Addison-Wesley Publishing Co.

Carkhuff, R. (1969a). *Helping and human relations, Vol. I: Selection and training.* New York: Holt, Rinehart and Winston.

Carkhuff, R. (1969b). *Helping and human relations, Vol. II: Practice and research.* New York: Holt, Rinehart and Winston.

Dagenais, F., & Meleis, A. I. (1982). Professionalism, work ethic, and empathy in nursing: The nurse self-description form. *Western Journal of Nursing Research, 4*, 407–422.

Duldt, B. (1981). Anger: An occupational hazard for nurses. *Nursing Outlook, 29*(9), 510–518.

Duldt B. (1982). Helping nurses cope with the anger–dismay syndrome. *Nursing Outlook, 30*(3), 168–175.

Duldt B. (1982). Helping nurses cope with the anger–dismay syndrome. *Nursing Outlook, 30*(3), 168–175.

Farrell, M., Haley, M., & Magnasco, J. (1977). Teaching interpersonal skills. *Nursing Outlook, 25,* 322–325.

Gagan, J. M. (1983). Methodological notes on empathy. *Advances in Nursing Science, 5*(2), 65–72.

Gazda, G. M., Childers, W. C., & Walters, R. P. (1982). *Interpersonal communication: A handbook for health professionals.* Rockville, MD: Aspen.

Gazda, G. M., Walters, R. P., & Childers, W. C. (1975). *Human relations development.* Boston: Allyn and Bacon.

Graffam, S. R. (1970). Nurse response to the patient in distress—development of an instrument. *Nursing Research, 19,* 331–336.

Kalisch, B. J. (1971). An experiment in the development of empathy in nursing students. *Nursing Research, 20,* 202–211.

Kelly, L. Y. (1981). *Dimensions of professional nursing* (4th ed.). New York: Macmillan.

Lambert, M. (1982). Relation of helping skills to treatment outcome. In E. K. Marshall & P. D. Kurtz, & Associates (Eds.), *Interpersonal helping-skills* (pp. 26–53). San Francisco: Jossey-Bass.

La Monica, E. L. (1981). Construct validity of an empathy instrument. *Research in Nursing and Health, 4,* 389–400.

La Monica, E. L. (1983). Empathy can be learned. *Nursing Education, 8*(2), 19–23.

La Monica, E. L., Carew, D. K., Winder, A. E., Haase, A. M. B., & Blanchard, K. H. (1976). Empathy training as a major thrust of a staff development program. *Nursing Research, 25,* 447–451.

La Monica, E. L., & Karshmer, J. (1978). Empathy: Educating nurses in professional practice. *Journal of Nursing Education, 17,* 3–11.

La Monica, E. L., Madea, A. R., & Oberst, M. T. (1987). Empathy and nursing care outcomes. *Scholarly Inquiry for Nursing Practice: An International Journal, 1*(3), 197–213.

Layton, J. M. (1978). *The use of modeling to teach empathy to nursing students.* Unpublished doctoral dissertation, Michigan State University, Ann Arbor, Michigan.

Layton, J. M. (1979). The use of modeling to teach empathy to nursing students. *Research in Nursing and Health, 2,* 163–176.

Morton, T. D., & Kurtz, P. D. (1982). Conditions affecting skills learning. In E. K. Marshall, P. D. Kurtz, & Associates (Eds.), *Interpersonal helping skills* (pp. 394–422). San Francisco: Jossey-Bass.

Omery, A. (1983). Moral development: A differential evaluation of dominant models. *Advances in Nursing Science, 6*(1), 1–17.

Payne, P. A., Weiss, S. D., & Kapp, R. A. (1972). Didactic, experiential, and modeling factors in the learning of empathy. *Journal of Counseling Psychology, 19,* 425–429.

Peitchinis, J. A. (1972). Therapeutic effectiveness of counseling by nursing personnel. *Nursing Research, 21,* 138–148.

Peitchinis, J. A. (1976). *Staff–patient communication in the health services.* New York: Springer Publishing Company.

Perry, M. A. (1975). Modeling and instruction in training for counselor empathy. *Journal of Counseling Psychology, 22,* 173–179.

Rogers, I. A. (1986). The effects of undergraduate nursing education on empathy. *Western Journal of Nursing Research, 8*(3), 329–342.

Steibe, S. C., Boulet, D. B., & Lee, D. C. (1979). Trainee trait empathy, age, trainer functioning, client age and training time as discriminators of successful empathy training. *Canadian Counsellor, 14*(1), 41–46.

Stetler, C. B. (1977). Relationship of perceived empathy to nurses' communication. *Nursing Research, 26,* 432–438.

Sundeen, S. J., Stuart, G. W., Rankin, E. D., & Cohen, S. A. (1985). *Nurse-patient interaction* (3rd ed.). St. Louis: C. V. Mosby.

Williamson-Kirkland, T. E., & Williamson-Kirkland, R. H. (1980). Teaching communication skills in rehabilitation medicine. *Archives of Physical Medicine and Rehabilitation, 61,* 221–224.

9

The Professional's Use of Empathy and Client Care Outcomes

Ruth C. MacKay
E. Joyce Carver
Jean R. Hughes

The first section of this chapter discusses the findings reported in the literature concerning the professional's use of empathy on client outcomes. The second section describes our study of the relationship between nurses' use of empathy and patient self-disclosures in the Burn and Plastic Surgery Unit.

REPORTED FINDINGS OF EMPATHY ON CLIENT OUTCOMES

The research literature describing the effects of the professional's use of empathy on client outcomes is based on three different approaches: (a) empathy as it affects the helping behavior of someone exposed to a person in need, (b) empathy as it may influence client self-disclosures, which in turn may affect client care, and (c) empathy as it affects various outcomes of professional care.

Empathy and Helping Behavior

Most of the studies reviewed concerning empathy and helping behavior are laboratory experiments in which empathy is manipulated as the experimental variable, and helping behavior in some sort of context is the observed outcome. A model put forth by Batson, Coke, and other colleagues (Batson, O'Quin, Fultz, & Vanderplas, 1983; Coke, Batson, & McDavis, 1978) places the study subject as observer of a person depicted to be in need. The empathic emotion engendered in the subject through taking the perspective of the observed other is reasoned to lead to helping behavior. Subjects in the manipulated high-empathy conditions were seen to offer more helping behavior than those in the low-empathy conditions (Barnett, Howard, King, & Dino, 1981). Moreover, easy or difficult escape from the helping situation separated subjects into those who showed altruistic helping behavior versus those who showed egoistic behavior to reduce their own distress (Toi & Batson, 1982). Namie (1982/1983), however, was not able to show significant results when rewards were used to influence helping; under reward conditions, emotional arousal was not seen to be influential in modifying helping behavior.

Other personality attributes may affect the empathy–helping relationship. Betancourt (1983) discussed a causal model in which the victim's need and the perspective adopted by the helper affect helping, with perceived controllability of the attribution of need exerting a significant influence. Davis (1983) has argued that empathy affects helping behavior in complex ways, with a number of variables in a multidimensional view of empathy influencing the helping outcome.

Watson, Hood, Morris, and Hall (1984) studied religious orientation as it is associated with empathy as a personality dimension. Their findings suggest that intrinsic religiosity, "viewing religion as the central 'end' around which life is organized" (p. 211) is directly related to empathy, and that extrinsic religiosity, "employing religion as a 'means' to selfish ends" (p. 211) is inversely related to empathy. The investigators suggest that empathic motivation may explain some of the relationship between religiosity and helping behavior (p. 215).

Empathic motivation and propensity to help are active areas of research. The few studies cited here give a sample of only some of the findings within these fields of study. As yet, however, the link between propensity to help and the effect of help on client outcomes has yet to be established.

Davitz and Davitz (1981) studied nurses' inferences of patients' pain and psychological distress. During their several studies they identified ten nurses who appeared to give nursing care which "was composed of something more than efficiency, knowledge, and technical skills" (p. 85). Interviews of these nurses revealed them to be exceptional in terms of commitment to nursing, confidence in their abilities, both as a person and as a professional, and a caring attitude to the patient. They recommended further study to ascertain the impact of what they termed is the empathic nurse on patients, and for the preparation of nurses who are rated high on empathy (pp. 85–100).

Empathy and Client Self-disclosures

The client's willingness to make self-disclosures to the helping professional has been linked to helper skill in interpersonal communication in a number of studies (Carkhuff, 1969; Truax & Carkhuff, 1967, pp. 159–161). The findings across studies, however, are not consistent. Newell (1979/1980) was unable to support the hypothesis that therapist empathy was related to frequency of client self-disclosures. Rockers (1976/1977) also found that interviewees did not alter significantly the amount of data disclosed in an initial history-taking interview when the mode of interviewing, using an open or closed form of questioning, was varied.

Dawson, Schirmer, and Beck (1984) reported the perception of clinician empathy to be positively related to patient reports of willingness to disclose information about health care to their health care providers (p. 143). In a subsequent study, Dawson (1985) found that patients with hypertension were different from other patients. They perceived less empathy in clinicians, and attributed greater importance to discussing with their health care provider their responses to health care, as compared with personal problems and lifestyle matters.

Empathy and Client Outcomes

The largest number of reported studies of empathy in helper–client interaction comes from the field of counseling and psychotherapy. Carkhuff and his associates cite several studies demonstrating the positive effects of facilitative communication (which includes empathy as one core dimension) on client self-exploration, client termination of therapy, and student academic achievement (Carkhuff, 1969, Vol. II, pp. 291–301). These and other studies by this same group have been reviewed by Lambert and DeJulio (1977), who raise serious questions about the methods used in the various studies, claiming that the evidence given for positive client outcomes cannot be accepted as conclusive.

Gladstein (1977) analyzed 18 studies reporting outcomes of psychotherapy as distinct from counseling. He summarized the evidence, stating that empathy was related to positive psychotherapy outcomes (such as in improved adjustment), and that empathy was not related clearly to positive client outcome when offered by counselors. In line with Gladstein's analysis, Truax, Wittmer, and Wargo (1971) reported effects of high empathy on positive personality changes of schizophrenic patients. In contrast, Mullen and Abeles (1971) found high empathy to be related to successful outcome of clients of counselors in a college setting, as evidenced by changes in scores on the Minnesota Multiphasic Personality Inventory clinical scales.

More recently, Valle (1981) studied the influence of counselor interpersonal functioning, that is, skills in the use of empathy, genuineness, respect, and concreteness, on the outcomes of clients receiving treatment for alcoholism. Higher levels of skills in counselors were associated with fewer relapse days over two years after treatment, fewer relapses, and less use of alcohol.

Three nursing studies give preliminary evidence that the nurse's use of empathy makes a difference in client outcomes. Williams (1979) stated that the level of empathy used by two nurse therapists was associated significantly with changes in self-concept of institutionalized elderly patients in group therapy over a period of eight weeks. The small sample size suggests caution in interpreting the results. Nonetheless the results are in agreement with Valle's findings with counselors, cited previously. Blackburn (1982/1983) reported sophomore nursing students who received training in empathic understanding in human relations to have higher ratings in clinical performance. Although clinical performance is not associated directly with client outcomes, there is an inferred relationship, not addressed empirically by Blackburn. La Monica, Wolf, Madea, and Oberst (1987) measured the effects of nurses' empathy before and after an empathy training program on the anxiety, depression, hostility and satisfaction with care of patients with cancer. They found less patient anxiety and hostility with patients cared for by nurses who had received the empathy training.

Review of the literature shows that research on the effects of empathic communication on client outcomes is sparse. As well, some studies show conflicting results. For many helping professionals, such as nurses, contacts with any one client may be limited in number and brief in duration, such as in an Emergency Department. It is difficult to assess the effects of empathy on clients when contact is short, disjointed, lacks continuity, or is shared with other helping professionals. Nonetheless, the cumulative influence of empathy from such interactions may be significant to the experience of clients. As well, there is little environmental control in many client settings, such as hospitals, where factors like privacy, noise, and interruptions from others must be considered. It must be concluded that the relationship between the professional's use of empathy and client wellbeing is as yet not fully explored, and that further research is in order.

INVESTIGATING NURSES' USE OF EMPATHY ON PATIENT SELF-DISCLOSURES

Client wellbeing is an outcome which can be expected to result from a number of factors, factors stemming from the nurses and clients themselves, from the environment in which the interaction transpires, and from the presenting client situation and treatment–care regimen. This has been discussed in Chapter 6. Nurses who assist clients to disclose information pertinent to their concerns and to their health are in a position to plan care which is directed to ameliorating problems related to health, and thus to facilitate recovery. The objective of the investigation reported here was to examine the relationship between the nurses' use of empathy and the self-disclosures of patients hospitalized for burns and other trauma.

We use La Monica's (1981) definition of empathy as, "accurate perception of the client's world by the helper, communication of this understanding to the client, and the client's perception of the helper's understanding" (p. 398).

Client disclosures are defined in a number of ways. Cozby (1973) states that self-disclosures are any information one person commu-

nicates verbally to another (p. 73). Adler (1973) distinguishes between self-disclosures and self-descriptions, stating that self-disclosures are a narrow subclass of self-descriptions which, in general, communicate motives. Cozby (1973), in reviewing the literature on self-disclosure, found the concept to be viewed in three
ways: (a) as a personality attribute, (b) as a component in interpersonal relationships, and (c) as examined in relation to nonverbal
aspects of communication. In our study, client disclosures, of
which self-disclosures are a subclass, can be defined as audible
revelations a client makes while in interaction with the helping
professional.

Method

There were 35 nurse-patient pairs who were observed during a
dressing change. Twelve nurses, all female, participated; five had a
diploma education, four had additional nursing education beyond
the diploma, and three had a baccalaureate degree in nursing.
Seven of the nurses had completed the empathy training program
described in Chapter 8. There were six male and three female
patients with education ranging from grade 5 to six years at a
university. All subjects volunteered to participate, and the interaction observed was pre-planned to occur at a time convenient to all
involved. The interactions were tape recorded and later transcribed. Both the tapes and transcripts were used simultaneously
in the analyses which followed.

Instrumentation

Empathy

Nurse responses to clients were rated using a modified version of
the scale published by Gazda, Walters, and Childers (1975, p. 246)
given in Chapter 5. Modifications were directed to establishing
more specific behavioral referents for each scale category, with an
accompanying set of rules for use of the scale. Although the 7-
point empathy scale was used in rating empathy, scores later were
collapsed into four categories, prompted by the distribution of
scores, namely: Level 1.0 (low), Level 2.0, Level 2.5, and Level 3.0
and higher (facilitative). Interrater agreement in identifying the
units of measurement (a nurse statement within the nurse's re-

sponse to the patient) was found to be 95 percent. Interrater reliability in categorizing these statements using the modified Empathy Scale was estimated to be .80 using Scott's Coefficient of Agreement.

The Self-Disclosure Category System

Four categories of patient disclosure were identified inductively from the recorded patient responses in this study and developed into a Self-Disclosure Category System. The entire response of the patient was divided first into units of disclosure for coding, and then each unit was classified in one of the four categories listed below.

Defensive self-disclosures

(Coded 1) include patient responses which are an appeal to be acknowledged by the nurse or which justify behavior. The category encompasses protective tactics to the self.

Content statement disclosures

(Coded 2) provide information for the nurse or ask questions. They maintain conversation through the offering of factual material.

Feeling disclosures

(Coded 3) verify patient feelings identified by the nurse. They do not reveal anything more of the self than what had originally been offered.

Volunteered self-disclosures

(Coded 4) are patient responses characterized by open communication in which personal information is volunteered by the patient. They confirm and extend revelations about the self and show the patient's emotional investment in the interaction.

Patient disclosures from the recorded interaction were rated in relation to what the nurse said to the patient in the prior exchange. There were separate ratings for each statement the patient made in the response. Interrater agreement by two raters in identifying the units of patient self-disclosure for classification was shown to be 93 percent. Scott's Coefficient of Agreement was computed to be .80 in classifying the units.

Analyses

Does the level of empathy which the nurse uses influence the quality of patient self-disclosure? Because patients and nurses were involved in more than one interaction each, a limitation of this study, a Spearman-Brown correlation coefficient was computed to assess separately the relationship between empathy statements and patient self-disclosures for each interaction episode (the period of observed interaction of one nurse–patient dyad). When there was more than one self-disclosure unit in the patient's response following the nurse's statement, the average self-disclosure rating was used for the analysis. There were 35 observed nurse–patient interactions. This analysis produced 35 coefficients with a mean of .16, ranging in value from $-.30$ to .36. Although the correlations were low, there is indication that higher levels of empathy were associated with the patient's volunteered disclosures. However, the examination of the relationship is obscured by the overwhelming number of nurse responses (70.9 percent) in which empathy is rated as 2.0, typically characterized by the nurse asking questions or giving information, with no attention to patient feelings and their meaning. Removing units in which empathy was rated as 2.0 from the analysis gave 13 interaction episodes in which the Spearman-Brown correlation coefficient was significant, with probabilities ranging from .05 to .003. The coefficients varied between .26 and .73 with a mean of .49. This shows that higher levels of nurse empathy were associated with more frequent use of patient self-disclosures.

Analyses of variance did not reveal that the nurses' clinical experience, education, or training in empathy skills influenced the values of these coefficients.

Selecting the highest rating of the nurse's use of empathy in each nurse-patient exchange, and analyzing this in relation to the highest rating of patient self-disclosure in that exchange (if there were multiple ratings), showed there to be a significant association. The analysis included all 35 interaction episodes, with 2.0 ratings of empathy omitted (see Table 9.1). A further analysis, using the same 35 interaction episodes and with empathy ratings of 2.0, revealed that the empathy training of nurses was significantly related to the nurse's use of higher levels of empathy ($\chi^2 = 11.9$, df $= 2$, $p = .003$).

It can be argued that perhaps some patients are more inclined to disclose information about themselves than others, reflecting

Table 9.1   Patient Disclosures by Nurse Empathy

Patient Disclosure Category	Nurse Empathy Ratings[a]		
	1 and 1.5	2.5	3 and 3.5
1	6	10	1
2	71	202	4
3	0	21	13
4	30	246	35
χ^2 = 89.68	df = 6	p < .0001	

Note: The highest ratings of empathy and self-disclosure in each nurse–patient exchange were selected if there were multiple ratings.
[a]2997 missing observations, including all empathy ratings of 2.0.

the influence of personality factors. Indeed, this was observed in the taped interactions. The possibility of this factor influencing the relationship of patient self-disclosures to the nurse's use of empathy was considered. Correlation coefficients derived from the same patient in different interactions were viewed to see if they were of similar size. The scattergram of size of coefficients by patient identity showed a random distribution, and no further analysis was undertaken, concluding that there was no observed effect in this small sample.

The analysis has indicated that nurses in dialogue with patients devote the major part of their interaction to concerns related to the giving of information and to the asking of questions, the empathy being rated as 2.0. These nurse responses do not acknowledge the affective dimension in the patients' statements. When empathy ratings at the higher and lower ends of the scale are viewed in relation to the patients' responses, a significant relationship between empathy and patient self-disclosures is uncovered. Higher levels of empathy are linked with greater frequencies of patient self-disclosures, and lower levels of empathy gave patient responses which were mainly factual in content, with feelings not revealed.

DISCUSSION

The most salient finding is the fact that 98 percent of nurse responses to the patient dealt only with factual material, without recognition of the affective dimension in the patient's message. This confirms what others have reported with both nurses and other helping professionals; the mean empathy rating is at a 2.0 level or below, indicating communication which is not facilitative (as examples see Carkhuff, 1969, Vol. I, pp. 154–155; Graffam, 1970; La Monica et al., 1976, p. 450; Layton, 1979, p. 168). The finding raises questions as to why such a large proportion of the nurse's dialogue fails to acknowledge the patient's stated or implied feelings. Several reasons can be suggested.

When a helping professional encourages the client to self-disclose, the professional may feel obligated to assist the client in managing associated emotions, or in some way intervene in the process of dealing with the problems which are disclosed. Not all helping professionals either are or feel confident or capable of doing so. These factors are discussed in some detail in chapters 8, 10, and 12 of this book.

The study reported here focused entirely on the interpretation of the transcribed dialogue between nurse and patient with only selected demographic factors introduced as modifiers of the relationship. Other factors, such as environmental constraints, may be important in explaining empathy, or empathy in relation to patient self-disclosures. Subsequent research in this area of practice needs to include additional factors.

CONCLUSIONS

The analysis has revealed that the quality of client self-disclosures was found to be associated with the level of empathy used by nurses as revealed in transcribed interactions. The lack of variability in the nurses' use of empathy, in which the large majority of ratings was found to be information-related, obscured and limited the examination of this variable. The training of nurses in the use of empathy was associated with higher levels of empathy in practice.

The small samples of nurses and patients are a limitation of this study as well. It is difficult to suggest, however, where there are enough nurses with high levels of empathy for study to permit the use of nurses once only in the sample. An experimental design using one nurse–client dyad, in which the level of empathy used is manipulated by a skilled practitioner, over time, might be one way of verifying the results reported here.

A further limitation of the study is the developmental state of the measure of self-disclosure. Continued study of the reliability and validity of the new category system is indicated.

The next chapter describes the qualitative analyses of the nurse–patient interaction discussed here, offering some validity to the quantitative analysis just reported.

REFERENCES

Adler, L. E. (1973). The dimensions of self-disclosure from three vantage points. (From *Dissertation Abstracts International*, 1973, *34*, Abstract No. 2294B.)

Barnett, M. A., Howard, J. A., King, L. M., & Dino, G. A. (1981). Helping behavior and the transfer of empathy. *Journal of Social Psychology*, *115*, 125–132.

Batson, C. D., O'Quin, K., Fultz, J., & Vanderplas, M. (1983). Influence of self-reported distress and empathy on egoistic versus altruistic motivation to help. *Journal of Personality and Social Psychology*, *45*, 706–718.

Betancourt, H. (1983). Causal attributions, empathy, and emotions as determinants of helping behavior: An integrative approach. (From *Dissertation Abstracts International*, 1983, *44*, Abstract No. 1636B.)

Blackburn, D. A. (1982/1983). The effect of human relations training on empathic understanding, self-concept and the clinical performance of sophomore student nurses. (From *Dissertation Abstracts International*, 1983, *43*, Abstract No. 2313B.)

Carkhuff, R. R. (1969). *Helping and human relations: A primer for lay and professional helpers*. Vols. I & II. New York: Holt, Rinehart & Winston.

Coke, J. S., Batson, C. D. & McDavis, K. (1978). Empathic mediation: A two-stage model. *Journal of Personality and Social Psychology*, *36* 752–766.

Cozby, P. C. (1973). Self-disclosure: A literature review. *Psychological Bulletin*, *79*, 73–91.

Davis, M. H. (1983). The effects of dispositional empathy on emotional reactions and helping: A multidimensional approach. *Journal of Personality*, *51*, 167–184.

Davitz, J. R., & Davitz, L. L. (1981). *Inferences of patients' pain and psychological distress*. New York: Springer Publishing Company.

Dawson, C. (1985). Hypertension, perceived clinician empathy, and patient self-disclosure. *Research in Nursing and Health*, *8*, 191–198.

Dawson, C., Schirmer, M., & Beck, L. (1984). A patient self-disclosure instrument. *Research in Nursing and Health*, *7*, 135–147.

Gazda, G. M., Walters, R. P., & Childers, W. C. (1975). *Human relations development*. Boston: Allyn & Bacon.

Gladstein, G. A. (1977). Empathy and counseling outcome: An empirical and conceptual review. The Counseling Psychologist, 6(4), 70–79.

Graffam, S. R. (1970). Nurse response to the patient in distress—Development of an instrument. Nursing Research, 19, 331–336.

Lambert, M. J., & DeJulio, S. S. (1977). Outcome research in Carkhuff's Human Resource Development Training Programs: Where is the donut? The Counseling Psychologist, 6(4), 79–86.

La Monica, E. L. (1981). Construct validity of an empathic instrument. Research in Nursing and Health, 4, 389–400.

La Monica, E. L., Carew, D. K., Winder, A. E., Haase, A. M. B., & Blanchard, K. H. (1976). Empathy training as a major thrust of a staff development program. Nursing Research, 25, 447–451.

La Monica, E. L., Wolf, R. M., Madea, A. R., & Oberst, M. T. (1987). Empathy and nursing care outcomes. Scholarly Inquiry for Nursing Practice: An International Journal, 1, 197–213.

Layton, J. M. (1979). The use of modeling to teach empathy to nursing students. Research in Nursing and Health, 2, 163–176.

Mullen, J., & Abeles, N. (1971). Relationship of liking, empathy, and therapist's experience to outcome of therapy. Journal of Counseling Psychology, 18, 39–43.

Namie, G. M. (1982/1983). Empathic and egoistic motivational bases of helping. (From Dissertation Abstracts International, 1983, 43, Abstract No. 2745B.)

Newell, M. E. (1979/1980). The effect of therapist empathy, norm disclosure, and self-disclosure on client self-disclosure and attraction to the therapist. (From Dissertation Abstracts International, 1980, 40, Abstract No. 3412B.)

Rockers, O. S. F. D. (1976/1977). The effects of open and closed inquiry modes used by counselors and physicians in an initial interview on interviewee perceptions and self-disclosure. (From Dissertation Abstracts International, 37, Abstract No. 7548A–7549A.)

Toi, M., & Batson, C. D. (1982). More evidence that empathy is a source of altruistic motivation. Journal of Personality and Social Psychology, 43, 281–292.

Truax, C. B., & Carkhuff, R. R. (1967). Toward effective counseling and pychotherapy: Training and practice. Chicago: Aldine.

Truax, C. B., Wittmer, J., & Wargo, D. G. (1971). Effects of the therapeutic conditions of accurate empathy, non-possessive warmth, and genuineness on hospitalized mental patients during group therapy. Journal of Clinical Psychology, 27, 137–142.

Valle, S. K. (1981). Interpersonal functioning of alcoholism counselors and treatment outcome. Journal of Studies on Alcohol, 42, 783–790.

Watson, P. J., Hood, R.W., Jr., Morris, R. J., & Hall, J. R. (1984). Empathy, religious orientation, and social desirability. Journal of Psychology, 117, 211–216.

Williams, C. L. (1979). Empathic communication and its effect on client outcome. *Issues in Mental Health Nursing*, 2(1), 15–26.

AUTHORS' NOTES

The research reported here was presented in part at the International Nursing Research Conference, Edmonton, Alberta, Canada, May 7, 1986, and at the Third Open Conference of the Workgroup of European Nurse-Researchers, Helsinki, Finland, August 15, 1986.

10

The Effects of Empathy on the Dynamics of Professional–Patient Interaction

Jean R. Hughes
E. Joyce Carver

This chapter reports the effects of nurse empathy on the content and process features of conversation during 35 recorded nurse-patient interactions. Two methods were used to determine the effects of empathy: (a) a content analysis of subject matter discussed and (b) a comparative analysis of selected case studies. Each method and the findings are discussed in turn.

CONTENT ANALYSIS

A content analysis of 35 nurse-patient conversations was conducted to describe the recurrent themes discussed and to determine how the discussions varied when nurses used facilitative empathy. The analysis began with two researchers grouping transcribed items of content into broad categories which were further defined and collapsed in accordance with established approaches described by Wilson (1985, p. 408). Content validity was checked with two outside researchers.

The unit of analysis was the complete nurse or patient statement. The units were rated in sequence and previous statements were used to determine the context. However, when a clear change of topic occurred within any unit and more than one content area was present, each topic was categorized. The two researchers achieved an interrater reliability of .87 using Scott's coefficient of agreement for categorizing the content in a sample of three transcripts.

The content categories together with the central question each addressed are listed below, and their descriptive criteria are discussed in sequence:

1. Healing Process: "Am I getting better?"
2. Wound care: "How do we do this?"
3. Coping: "How will I get through this?"
4. Feelings: "How do I feel?"
5. Significant others: "How are they getting along?"

Conversations related to the *healing process* explored experiences associated with the condition and treatment of the wound. Information focused on the progress made over time, including what had happened to the wound, how it was now, and what it might be like in the future. The conversation considered the following factors: the appearance of the wound and how it would change (color, size, drainage, scabs/blisters, swelling, circulation, temperature); tests, surgery, treatments, procedures, and exercises; the progression of treatment activities including physician plans and what the physician had told the patient; the results of tests; and the anticipated length of hospital stay, discharge plans, and follow-up treatment.

Wound care discussion centered on the here and now as it related to the logistics of the dressing change. Discussion included the type of dressing and materials used; the timing, location, and procedure employed for the dressing change; positioning and preparations for the event; explanations/information about the solutions/materials used, and what to expect as the dressing change proceeded.

Coping conversation addressed those physical activities and mental mechanisms generated to accommodate the injury. Specific strategies were identified which helped patients or nurses survive the stressful ordeal and gain control over aspects of care. These focused on assuming control of aspects of treatment to endure the hurt (e.g., where to begin the dressing), pain management and medication, physical accommodation (e.g., gritting teeth), commitment to treatment as evidenced by what the patient was willing to do, reviewing the accident or circumstances surrounding the injury in graphic detail, comparing progress to that of other patients; defense mechanisms (e.g., sarcasm, rationalization), approval giving or seeking, and reviewing the patient's related past experiences or knowledge.

Feelings discussion focused on the physical sensations and emotional reactions to the injury, treatment, and recovery process. Physical sensations included the characteristics and location of the pain or discomfort, and all other bodily feelings such as itching, numbness, tickling, or burning. Emotional reactions encompassed explicitly verbalized worries/concerns either present or anticipated, such as worry about the meaning of changes in wound appearance, anxiety about imminent surgery, fear of possible infection, and feelings related to hospitalization.

Conversation related to *Significant others* discussed the effects of the patient's illness on family, relatives, and friends and referred to their visits, their phone calls, their well-being, and their activities or reactions related to the injury.

Findings

Slightly more than one-half of all conversation in the 35 interactions centered on Healing process and Wound care (Table 10.1). Coping was the third-largest category and content about Significant others occurred least frequently. There were numerous miscellaneous items which did not fit into the five designated categories, such as, social chit-chat about the weather or television programs and comments about the environment. These were unrelated to patient care. As the varied topics seemed inconsequential in context, they were therefore not included in the analysis. It is interesting to note, however, that light chit-chat formed 10 percent of the subject matter discussed.

Feelings were discussed 14 percent of the time and the majority of this content was about physical sensations (Table 10.2).

Although only 4 percent of the content was about specifically

Table 10.1   Subject Matter Discussed During a Dressing Change
(N = 35)

Content category	M[a]	SD	Range
Healing process	28.77[b]	13.24	6–60
Wound care	23.43	15.07	2–63
Coping	19.23	10.06	3–43
Feelings	14.20	6.44	3–31
Significant others	3.71	4.95	0–18

[a]Mean of percent of total for each interaction.
[b]Column total < 100 because miscellaneous subject matter was discarded.

stated emotional concerns, patient statements which fell in the other categories often alluded to anxieties about getting better. Emotions were directly labeled by the patient or nurse in 26 or 74.3 percent of the 35 interactions. Nine interactions lacked any direct mention of feeling words by either party.

It became evident that patients focused their statements primarily on their concerns about getting better, but these were indirectly expressed the majority of the time. Gazda, Childers & Walters (1982) note that the first things patients mention are usually not the most important to them and that patients often mask their requests for understanding. Furthermore, patients may conceal their needs and test the professional's response as they gradually work toward discussion of sensitive topics. This allows patients to pull back if they find the professional is not understanding (Gazda, Childers & Walters, 1982, pp. 58–59). Although they were seldom expressed openly, powerful feelings seemed to lurk at the core of most discussions as patients cautiously searched for empathy from the nurse.

Discussions about wound care were factual and distinctly differ-

Table 10.2   Sub-groupings of Subject Matter in the Feelings Category
(N = 35)

Feelings	M[a]	SD	Range
Physical sensations	10.26	5.52	2–24
Emotional concerns	3.94	4.16	0–19
Total	14.20	6.44	3–31

[a]Mean of percent of total for each interaction.

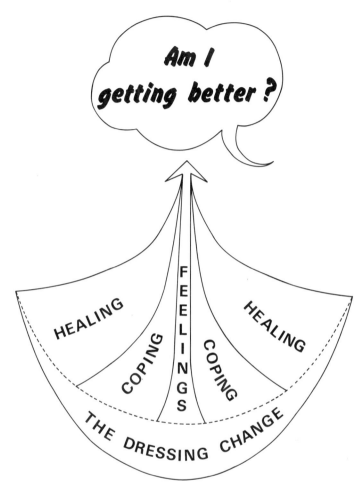

FIGURE 10.1   The focus of nurse–patient conversation during a dressing change.

ent in nature from conversations about coping and healing. The latter often contained an undercurrent of patient worries.

Emotional feelings were concealed like the innermost layers of an onion. Discussion about coping and the healing process could be visualized as the outer, surface layers which formed the most frequent, more general, and least threatening topics of conversation. A wellspring of feeling lay at the center. Except for task-related content about wound care, most of the dialogue was aimed at the overall patient concern, "Am I getting better?" The following example illustrates this:

> P: I've never seen the crater on the other side [of my foot]. It's just like being on the other side of the moon.
>
> N: Well, actually the other side is a little bit bigger than this, and it's not a crater, it's just that the skin is necrotic, like it's very dark looking, and it's about the size of a fifty-cent piece.
>
> P: Oh well, that's not quite so ominous as it was at first.
>
> N: And it's not deep, it's close to the surface.
>
> P: Oh well, maybe I'll get away with just losing [by surgery] a toe after all.

Here the patient's request for information about the wound's appearance emanated from fear about the extent of potential surgical treatment.

Relationship to the Nurse's Use of Facilitative Empathy

Further data analysis was done to determine how the topics discussed during the dressing change varied when the nurse's responses included facilitative empathy (level three or above). Nurses used no facilitative empathy in 16 interactions. In the remaining 19 cases the nurse's use of facilitative empathy was not extensive, with a range of 1–7 responses per interaction and a mode of 1 empathy response per interaction (Table 10.3).

Table 10.3   Number of Facilitative Empathic Responses by Interaction

No. of empathy responses in interaction f	Interactions $N = 35$	Total no. of empathy responses $N = 59$
0	16	0
1	6	6
2	4	8
3	1	3
4	2	8
5	3	15
6	2	12
7	1	7

NOTE: Empathy refers to facilitative, level 3 or above, responses as described in Chapter 5.

The total number of level 3 empathic responses was limited to 59 in the 35 interactions. Nurses who used facilitative empathy tended to discuss the logistics of wound care only to the extent necessary to accomplish the task at hand, or to answer direct questions. Instead the nurse and patient talked more about emotional concerns and coping.

COMPARATIVE CASE STUDY ANALYSIS

Following the description of nurse–patient conversations in terms of content characteristics, a comparative case-study analysis (Wilson, 1985, pp. 136–138; Strauss & Glasser, 1970) was conducted to examine the same interactions in relation to process features. Rawnsley (1987) supports this approach and cautions investigators about examining empathy purely as a quantitative construct. She suggests that the "dynamic, interactive properties" (p. 218) are critical elements requiring qualitative analysis as well.

It is recognized that qualitative analysis of conversation can expose an individual in a more personal way than many other methods. We commend the nurses who allowed us to observe their interactions with patients. We believe the strengths and limitations identified in the verbal performance are most likely not unique to this population may help to explain the complexity of professional–client interaction of use to the development of nursing as one of the caring professions.

The 35 transcriptions were reviewed first according to nurse-empathy frequency counts and then according to issue and process features. Based on the above, they were identified as being predominantly level 1, 2, or 3 empathy interactions. Content validity and a two-step reliability check were independently conducted by two investigators. This review resulted in complete agreement with the (a) description of process and issue features, (b) classification of each of the interactions for level of empathy according to process features, (c) classification of interactions for level of empathy according to their nurse-empathy frequency counts, and (d) interclassification of interactions for level of empathy according to (b) and (c) above.

The dynamics that occurred in level 1, 2, and 3 empathy interactions were addressed in terms of the following issues which surfaced in all conversations:

1. Sequencing: The degree of purposeful progression of the interaction.
2. Control: Who controlled the conversation.
3. Focus: The nature of the subject matter.

Level One Case Studies

Level one empathy can be summarized to include reponses that reflect irrelevant or hurtful remarks that do not appropriately attend to the surface feelings of the patient (Gazda et al., 1982).

Sequencing

These interactions were not progressive and demarcation between phases was absent. The beginning stage of the interaction failed to include an introduction, setting of expectations, and preliminary exploration of patient concerns as suggested by the literature (see for example Gazda et al. 1982; Northouse & Northouse, 1985; Sundeen, Stuart, Rankin, & Cohen, 1985). Presumably the only indication the patient had that a dressing change would occur was by the presence of tangible, familiar equipment.

The middle phase of an effective interaction typically involves a specific, focused inquiry that follows logically from the issues raised during the exploration stage of the interview (see for example Gazda et al., 1982; Northouse & Northouse, 1985; Sundeen et al., 1985). However, these middle-phase discussions were disjointed and occurred in isolated segments, reflecting the same superficial tone established earlier. Rapport was not developed, and the parties gained little mutual understanding as they appeared unable to follow the basic theme of conversation.

The final phase of an ideal interaction capitalizes on the foundations established in the beginning and works toward decision-making or resolution of problems (see for example Gazda et al., 1982; Northouse & Northouse, 1985; Sundeen et al., 1985). However, in the later stages of the level one interactions, goals could not be achieved as issues had not been mutually recognized, expectations were absent and therefore action was impossible. The nurse queried the patient in an imposing manner, perhaps to maintain control over the situation. Closure was not attempted. Both nurse and patient merely drifted apart as the nurse signaled the end of the conversation for example, by gathering up her equipment and leaving the patient's room.

Control

These interactions provided a clear demonstration of how professionals can manipulate conversations, probably unconsciously, to suit their own needs. Without being unpleasant the nurse enforced her wishes by simply not addressing specific patient concerns.

The major control feature in this interaction was the persistent use of questions. In general, Gazda and his colleagues (1982) believe "the greater number of questions, the less likelihood that the helper can assist" (p. 171). They acknowledge the appropriateness of inquiry when it is employed to obtain objective data, to clarify, or to pinpoint information (pp. 168–169). However, many of the questions in these interactions lacked apparent purpose and continuity, and therefore answers would be unlikely to assist the nurse in gaining an understanding of the patient's world. This creates heightened tension for the patient as the questions reduce rather than facilitate self-exploration, and the patient becomes discouraged from volunteering what might be judged by the nurse as irrelevant information (p. 170).

Close examination shows that questions were often asked when the answers were already or should have been known. Commonly requested information, for example about whether the patient had the dressing done before, would be available on the patient's chart and should be a part of the routine preparation carried out prior to giving nursing care. The presence of these types of questions can be interpreted to mean that *either* the nurse had not prepared herself regarding patient progress before entering the room *or* that the questions were asked to fill a silence. The fact that the nurse frequently did not pursue a subject once the patient answered the initial question lends support to the latter explanation.

The nurse initiated new topics of conversation almost exclusively. The subjects chosen by the patient referred to safe content in which the patient had to invest little. On the occasions the patient disclosed some personal information about ideas, feelings, or reactions, the nurse usually changed the subject following the patient's disclosure. For example, when a patient commented, "I had to have some great big person needling in my groin." the nurse responded, "Is the Dakin's [solution] stinging [your toe wound] at all?" Changing topics is a nontherapeutic technique that puts the nurse in charge of material discussed" (Sundeen et al., 1985, p. 124). The practice is often used as a means of protection from anxiety-laden issues. The tension could result from a failure to listen, or a belief that the patient is incapable of helping himself and therefore not able to select appropriate topics for discussion (Sundeen et al., 1985, p. 124).

As subject matter changed frequently patients, whose injuries placed them in vulnerable positions, may have felt even more unsure of what behaviors were expected of them. Teamwork did not exist in these interactions. Rather, participants appeared to be isolated, and a clear direction was not indicated for many of the conversations. Patients appeared to adopt a cautious attitude and assume a subordinate role perhaps thinking that if they were compliant the authority figure would provide them with solutions (Gazda et al., 1982, p. 169). Such expectations generally were unfulfilled.

Focus

Consistent with the findings of the content analysis, the nurse effectively maintained the focus on objective information while failing to respond to cues related to abstract issues during level one interactions. The subject matter was given little attention, often became disjointed and appeared confusing for the patient as indicated by frequent requests for the nurse to repeat comments. Conversations most frequently addressed issues considered to be of a miscellaneous, non-focused nature. Matters of wound care, relating to the logistics of the dressing change, were discussed to a lesser extent during these interactions. Only minimal attention was given to abstract information concerning coping stategies or feelings experienced, including physical sensations and emotions.

Inference

It can be concluded that level one empathy interaction centered on the nurse's need to complete a task with little acknowledgement of the patient's personal world or the need for patient involvement.

Level Two Empathy Case Studies

Level two empathy can be summarized to incorporate accurate content, either in a general or more specific format. It enables nurses and patients to work in relative harmony but does not contain a verbal reflection of patient feelings.

Sequencing

The sequencing of these conversions was progressive in that the patient revealed more personal information as the conversation progressed. However, a clear distinction between phases of the interaction was not entirely obvious.

The conversations began in a somewhat similar manner as that depicted with level one empathy. The dressing change started immediately without an introduction or expectations being established. Perhaps the participants had learned role expectations from previous encounters, since both parties appeared to understand the other's thoughts and seemed willing to concentrate on the task at hand. A degree of harmony was present.

During the middle phase the interaction became somewhat less superficial. The nurse provided explanations with her answers to patient inquiries and gave accurate responses without false reassurance. In facilitative interactions the goal of the middle phase is to achieve understanding of the patient care situation (Gazda et al., 1982). These conversations contained the essential elements to make this possible. This is in contrast to level one case studies where the nurse and patient appeared to work together only when the conversation moved to a neutral subject which was unrelated to patient care.

The final phase of level two interaction provided little difference from level one case studies. The nurse began to distance herself by giving superficial answers to the patient's questions without attending to the underlying messages. However, rather than leaving the room without verbal warning as in level one interaction, the nurse signaled her termination, for example by saying, "there" which can be interpreted to mean, "I'm finished."

Control

The level two interaction developed a sense of shared responsibility in which the nurse invited patient input. This involvement in the decisions concerning treatment may have helped the patient to experience greater control (Northouse & Northouse, 1985, pp. 41–45). On the occasions when the patient disclosed some personal information, the nurse pursued the subject. This reaction could be interpreted as a demonstration of respect for the patient's role in the interaction.

A feeling of teamwork did develop between parties; however, the nurse was clearly the dominant participant in that she initiated new topics much more frequently than the patient. Individuals often left parts of their thoughts unstated, but in contrast to the level one conversations, each seemed to understand the other's message. According to Gazda and his colleagues (1982) level two empathy communicates only partial awareness of patient surface feelings. It is generally a mechanical or reactive response, but the focus does remain on the patient. It would appear this partial awareness was sufficient to accomplish the fundamentals of the required task.

Focus

Approximately one-half of the conversation addressed wound care activities, and the technicalities of the healing process were discussed to a lesser extent. These findings are consistent with Clark's (1981) work. "For 75% of all NPC [nurse–patient communication] the substance of the conversation was related to aspects of treatment and care" (1981, p. 14). Only limited segments of the interaction focused on the psychosocial domains of feelings experienced and coping strategies, with emphasis on physical sensations rather than emotions. Sofaer (1984) states that "many nurses develop feelings of powerlessness and frustration when they are unable to relieve suffering and may blame themselves or others" (p. 76). It may be that nurses managed these unpleasant feelings by attending only to those aspects of patient care over which they had control. This was frequently demonstrated through the provision of concrete information. For example, one patient asked, "[My hair] won't grow in that part, will it?" to which the nurse replied, "It probably won't where the skin graft is."

Inference

These interactions were clearly not facilitative but neither were they hurtful. Their inoffensive nature might not have alerted *either* the patient *or* the nurse to interaction weaknesses. Therefore the nurse's skill deficits would unlikely be identified, and the relationship would continue without improvement.

Level Three Empathy Case Studies

Level three empathy conveys the message that the patient has been understood at the level being expressed and that surface feelings have been accurately reflected (Gazda et al., 1982). The focus of the conversation remains with the patient.

Sequence

The sequencing throughout these interactions was obvious with a clear distinction between phases. A progressively more intense relationship developed with each response.

In the beginning of these conversations the nurse inquired about the patient's thoughts. Such an approach establishes that the nurse is prepared to make a significant investment which in turn fosters a sense of safety about the professional (Collins, 1978; Gazda et al., 1982; Northouse & Northouse, 1985; Rogers, 1975; Sundeen et al., 1985). It recognizes that patients often need encouragement to disclose their feelings but that they may experience great relief "simply by being made to feel free to do this" (Sofaer, 1984, p. 75).

The nurse pursued the level three conversation with great sensitivity. She indicated her willingness to explore an issue in depth but remained attuned to patient cues that a change of subject was warranted. Trust begins to emerge as the patient "feels that another individual will behave in ways that are beneficial to the relationship, without attempting to control or direct it" (Northouse & Northouse, 1985, p. 45). "Losing control takes from clients a primary means of ascribing meaning to their lives" (Cantor cited in Northouse & Northouse, 1985, p. 41). The nurse in these interactions was careful to let the patient determine the direction of conversation. For example, during a discussion about the onset of an infection, the patient was distracted by thoughts of the impending dressing change and altered the topic with the comments, "I always hate this [dressing change]". Recognizing the pain–anxiety cycle (Black, 1987) that often accompanies a treatment procedure, the nurse responded to the patient's cue with her comment, "I know it's painful for you."

During the middle stage of an effective interaction the nurse and patient work on mutually agreed tasks. The relationship intensifies, becomes more comfortable, and a degree of predictability evolves (Sundeen et al., 1985, p. 184). These elements were present in level three interactions as the patient took risks and revealed personal worries. For example, one patient hinted that she had caused her infection. Many patients feel angry at themselves for causing or contributing to their injury, guilty for not taking more care, and resentful that the injury was a punishment

(Black, 1987, p. 450). In the above example the disclosure was respected as the nurse validated the patient's surface feelings and provided reassurance in her comments," Are you afraid that it might have been something that you had done that caused this? . . . I'm sure you always did your best to take care of it. It's just one of those things that happens."

It is during the middle phase that the nurse supports the understanding and development of coping mechanisms in the patient (Collins, 1978). For example, a patient asked, "Do you think it [the pain] gets worse as the day goes along?" To which the nurse replied, "Well it could be that. You know you're upset about it and you've seen it [the dressing change] done a couple of times and it's painful for you. So I can see by the end of the day you're feeling fed up and frustrated." This intervention encouraged the patient to develop insight and independent problem solving skills.

> During the encounter the person is discovering the realities of what is happening and what can be done about it, and this affects coping. . . . Learning that one lacks control over the most significant aspects of the situation will encourage the use of strategies for regulating emotions (Lazarus & Folkman, 1984, p. 148).

The final phase of the interaction affords opportunity for the evaluation of goal attainment and termination of the relationship/ visit (for example, Collins, 1978; Gazda et al., 1982; Hughes, 1985; Northouse & Northouse, 1985). For example, one nurse asked a patient directly for feedback, "How do you find the dressing?" and provided reassurance that it would remain secure. This same patient obviously trusted the nurse and conveyed a wish to maintain the relationship in her question, "Will you be doing it [the dressing] again? Will it be you?" "The satisfaction felt by both participants over having accomplished their mutual goals was balanced by the realization of the impending loss of a person with whom very meaningful experiences have been shared" (Sundeen et al., 1985, p. 194). As well, the patient's question demonstrates the anticipatory work that may be conducted so as to improve control over the situation. Lazarus and Folkman (1984) believe "The cognitive appraisal process evaluates whether, to what extent and how the person can manage the threat relevant to the sense of control . . . [the person may] look for information . . . on which other coping strategies might be predicted" (p. 145).

Control

Level three interactions displayed shared responsibility between the nurse and patient as they worked in collaboration to establish goals and expectations. Each responded to the other's cues and was comfortable raising issues of actual or potential concern, for mutual exploration. There did not appear to be any limitations regarding acceptable subject matter.

These interactions reflected differences in comparison to the level one and two empathy interactions. The patient generally initiated a new topic of conversation as often as the nurse, reflecting a much more equal distribution of control. Consistent with Begliner (cited in Geach, 1987, p. 544) the nurse was careful to inquire about, but not force, the patient's decisions.

The nurse rarely changed the subject following a patient disclosure. However, when alterations occurred they could be interpreted as therapeutic interventions, as in the case of moving the patient to a higher level of insight by introducing new and more sensitive information, or alerting the patient to the next step in the dressing change.

Focus

In contrast to level one and two interactions but consistent with the content analysis reported earlier, Level three concentrated on issues related to the psychosocial domain. Generally, more than half of the conversation related equally to coping strategies and feelings experienced, including physical sensations and emotions. The patient frequently volunteered information about private thoughts of a more personal nature than in level one and two interactions, and these revealed more specific content related to pain, fear of the dressing change, and attempts to manage discomfort.

Conversation seemed to accommodate factual content, related to the logistics of the dressing change and wound healing, as well as the abstract fears and painful responses to the necessary treatments. This division reflects a more balanced and holistic approach to interaction meeting both the physical and psychosocial needs of the patient.

Inference

Level three empathy showed movement toward mutually negotiated actions, a progressively more intimate relationship, as well as attention to both concrete and abstract subject matter. The commitment demonstrated by both parties to the pursuit of an effective relationship was clear, and it would appear the results of this collaborative effort achieved satisfaction for both the nurse and the patient.

SUMMARY

The foregoing analyses have provided an examination of content and process features reflected in interactions involving facilitative and non-facilitative nurse empathy. Clearly the dynamics of the discussion altered dramatically with varying degrees of nurse empathy. These qualitative analyses suggest support for the quantitative analyses regarding the positive influence of effective nurse empathy on patient well-being. However it is recognized that these results are tentative and further research is needed to clarify the dynamics of professional–patient interaction in relation to empathy.

REFERENCES

Black, J. (1987). Burns. In C. R. Kneisl and S. W. Ames (Eds.), *Adult health nursing: A biopsychosocial approach* (pp. 439–476). Menlo Park, CA: Addison-Wesley.

Clark, J. M. (1981). Communication in nursing. *Nursing Times, 77*(1), 12–18.

Collins, D. L. (1978). The one-to-one relationship. In L. A. Joel and D. L. Collins (Eds.), *Psychiatric nursing: Theory and application* (pp. 81–114). New York: McGraw-Hill.

Gazda, G. M., Childers, W. C., & Walters, R. P. (1982). *Interpersonal communication: A handbook for health professionals.* Rockville, MD: Aspen.

Geach, B. (1987). Coping with acute and chronic illness. In J. Norris, M. Kunes-Connell, S. Stockard, P. M. Ehrhart, and G. R. Newton (Eds.), *Mental health—psychiatric nursing: A continuum of care* (pp. 527–550). New York: John Wiley.

Hughes, J. (1985). Therapeutic use of self: The helping relationship, stress adaptation and crisis intervention. In M. Stewart, S. Searl, and C. Smillie (Eds.), *Community health nursing in Canada* (pp. 531–556). Toronto: Gage Publishing Company.

Lazarus, R. S., & Folkman, S. (1984). *Stress, appraisal and coping* (pp. 141–180). New York: Springer Publishing Company.

Northouse, P. G., & Northouse, L. L. (1985). Communication variables in health care. In *Health communication: A handbook for health professionals.* Englewood Cliffs, NJ: Prentice-Hall, Inc.

Rawnsley, M. M. (1987). Response to "Empathy and nursing care outcomes." *Scholarly Inquiry for Nursing Practice: An International Journal,* 1(3), 215–219.

Rogers, C. (1975). Empathic: An unappreciated way of being. *The Counselling Psychologist,* 5(2), 2–10.

Sofaer, B. (1984). *Pain: A handbook for nurses* (pp. 74–80). London: Harper & Row.

Strauss, A. L. & Glaser, B. G. (1970). Case histories and case studies. In *A case history of a dying trajectory anguish* (pp. 182–193). Mill Valley, CA: The Sociology Press.

Sundeen, S. J., Stuart, G. W., Rankin, E. D., & Cohen, S. A. (1985). *Nurse-client interaction: Implementing the nursing process.* 3rd edition. St. Louis: The C. V. Mosby Company.

Wilson, H. S. (1985). *Research in nursing.* Menlo Park, CA: Addison-Wesley.

ACKNOWLEDGMENT

The investigators acknowledge the skill and patience of Judy Murray in preparing the written transcript from the recorded interactions.

Part IV

The Challenges
of Applying Theory
to Practice

Earlier parts of the book have discussed conceptual orientations to empathy and investigations of empathy in relation to health care practice. Part Four describes some of the problems of putting empathy into professional practice.

Davis in Chapter 11 discusses cultural issues and the many pitfalls ready to catch unwary professionals communicating with those from cultures different from their own. Although his examples are drawn from nursing, the principles involved are pertinent to any field of health care practice.

Hughes and Carver in Chapter 12 focus on a number of specific problems which impede the professional's development of empathy skills, or which intrude on the use of these skills in the practice area. From their reading, experience, and the comments of students and practitioners alike, they put forward suggestions for overcoming some of these barriers to the use of facilitative empathy in practice.

Chapter 13 centers on seven issues concerning

the study of empathy and its importance to practice in the helping professions. What are the most pressing problems to be faced in promoting facilitative professional–client communication? What are the priorities for addressing these? Some suggestions are aired for future thought and deliberation.

11

Empathy in Transcultural Nursing Practice

Bryn D. Davis

Communication in helping relationships, in a multi-cultural setting, demands special consideration. It involves basic accurate empathy, which requires listening carefully to clients and then letting clients know that the emotional as well as the factual content of their stories is understood. If the story refers to experiences and situations, involving values and language which are very different from those of the helper, then the demonstration of empathy and respect which is fundamental to any helping relationship, requires a knowledge of cultural influences.

It is possible to identify several factors in transcultural helping relationships which need careful management in respect to practice. In the following sections of this Chapter we shall consider a) empathy in multicultural relationships, b) the social psychology of people's dealings with each other, c) self-image and its relationship to interactions with others, d) communication, and in particular, language, non-verbal communication, and emotional expression, e) client perceptions of the helper, f) helper's perceptions of the client, and g) the implications of these for helping in a transcultural context.

Helping relationships involve a variety of interacting pairs and groups. Because most nations are multicultural, either of longstanding or relatively recent development, there is need often for relationships which transcend cultural boundaries. Helping professionals may be members of the majority, with members of a minority or minorities as clients. Alternatively, they may be members of a minority with clients who are members of the majority or other minorities. The complexity of such multicultural relationships has been discussed elsewhere (Davis, 1986). Gender may also increase the complexity. Examples include situations where a Mauritian (first language French) is helping an Asian (first language Gujerati) through a common second language, English, or where a white male is helping a female Asian client. Also it may be difficult for a client who is from the dominant culture to accept that a helper from a very different minority culture can empathize accurately in that situation.

Most helping models incorporate a "bio-psychosocial" view of mankind into their attempts to generate a holistic approach to care, and this can be seen in practice on both sides of the Atlantic. However, there has recently been an increasing call for such models to include culture as well. This call has been particularly strong in North America, especially in the United States as revealed through the work of Leininger (1978) originally, but also Brink (1976), and Branch (1976). Without such a dimension in the model, it is argued, attempts to develop an empathic relationship may founder as a result of misperception of either verbal or non-verbal cues which have a strong cultural loading.

The concern for an ethnographic approach also has been expressed in the UK. Dobson (1983), for example, has recently completed a cross-cultural study in Scotland which was initially inspired by her experiences in Canada as a nurse. She has quoted Florence Nightingale as a source for her argument for cultural awareness in nurses (p. 56), but also notes the paucity of nursing literature supporting such an approach. The all-pervasive nature of cultural influences on behavior has been emphasized by Burrows (1983) as well, who claims that the current tendency to assume that all nurses and patients are from the same Christian, Caucasian culture can only be detrimental to quality care and must therefore change. When many members of the profession and of the society it serves are of a variety of cultures, such an ethos pervading the profession must limit the possibility of empathic approaches to care. In the counseling, psychotherapeutic, and helping relationships, understanding is the keystone, that is, understanding within the cultural context of both interacting partners.

EMPATHY IN MULTICULTURAL RELATIONSHIPS

Empathy can be defined as the ability to understand someone else's situation without making it one's own. Advanced empathy requires the ability to express an understanding of the unspoken, implied aspects of the client's story, to build bridges between sections of the story, expressed or implied, and to help the client to use these bridges in moving toward growth and development (Egan, 1986). The process of establishing rapport, and the facilitation of an exploration by clients of their situations, and reactions to them, are very difficult if not impossible to achieve (Egan, 1986). This level of understanding can occur only if the helper is able to "walk in the shoes" of the client. This kind of understanding therefore depends on the acceptance of cultural differences. True empathy offers this acceptance.

The accuracy of any empathy shown is judged by clients, of course. The meaning of their utterances, understood by the helper, are necessarily personal, although culture-bound. Thus clients have a view of the culture from which they come or within which they are living, which is similar to but different from others from that culture. It is not enough to know about a particular culture in general, although this can be useful at the beginning of a relationship. It is essential to know about a particular individual within a particular culture.

SOCIAL PSYCHOLOGY

The dynamics of interpersonal relationships, within which empathy is a central process, have been studied and many insights are now available to help practioners and their educators.

Models

When attempts are made to explain behavior, an expectation is offered based on what is already known or conjectured, and then tested for support in practice. These expectations are known as models.

Many psychologists believe that everyone uses models: of themselves, their relationships with others, and their culture in their everyday lives (e.g., Chapman & Jones, 1984; Kelly, 1955; Miller, Galanter, & Pibram, 1960). Different words are used to label these models, such as schema, constructs, and plans, but essentially they involve expectations about people or situations based on experience or other information. These expectations form the basis of our behavior with regard to ourselves or with others. If the expectation is valid and confirmed in reality, it stays, but if not it is usually modified or rejected in the light of the new information. This modification is the process of education, of therapy, or of general growth as an individual person.

A model of another person is usually based on first impressions, which can be potent determinants of our expectations of that person (see Brislin, 1981; and the discussion in Chapter 4 of this volume). They usually involve similarities and differences. The information gained is categorized, a process of organization where we give it personal meaning. The primacy of the information or its recency are very important, as is its salience or relevance to our self-image or self-esteem. This process of grouping or categorization very much simplifies the process of dealing with a lot of information about a lot of people, and as long as it facilitates social interaction, then it works. But it can lead to an oversimplification such that we deal not in realities but in stereotypes. In other words, we interact with others, not as individuals with personal idiosyncracies, but as representatives of a particular category of people.

Stereotypy

The grouping of others into simplistic categories relating to single attributes, which may often be physical, is a way in which people try to simplify the complexity of relationships. It can be also a way in which people avoid relationships where a real exchange of feelings and empathy is needed.

Stereotypy has been a focus of some concern in nurse–patient relationships for some time, and is the rationale for many of the models operating or being developed in order to retain the individuality of the patient and to facilitate empathic interactions (e.g., King, 1971; Peplau, 1952; Roy, 1970). Professionals in their practice have to try to overcome the natural processes of stereotypy in order that truly professional care for individual clients may be offered. See Davis (1984) for a discussion of this issue in more detail than can be covered here. There is strong evidence that nurses do have a tendency to deal with the average patient rather than the individual, particularly with reference to the assessment of stress experienced by patients (Johnston, 1976). Even though taking into account some of the psychosocial information often gained in patient assessment, the patient tends to be dealt with as "elderly," or "anxious" without any personal qualification, (see also Kelly & May, 1982).

The question of stereotypy, and the kind of attributions about people and their behavior in the transcultural context that result, have been discussed by Brislin (1981) in general social situations, and by Littlewood and Lipsedge (1982) and Rack (1982), in relation to mental health. Attributions are explanations of behavior, our own or others. Early researchers in the field (Jones & Davis, 1965) identified the fundamental attribution error as being the attribution of trait or type to the behavior of others, and of situational influence for self.

Attributions also include judgements about emotional states as well as personality traits. If attributions of feelings, or reactions to experiences are made in a stereotypical fashion (i.e., as for a particular "type" or "case") then any hope for an empathic relationship must be dashed. Showing empathy is in effect offering a model of someone's behavior for them to validate. Accurate empathy is an attribution of a particular characteristic that immediately locates and emphasizes the individual's unique experiences.

A major attribution that is made about others is that of belonging to an "in-group" or an "out-group", or to the "we" group or the "they" group. As Pocock (1975) argues, the more entrenched the "we", group, the more it is the majority, then the more likely it is to see itself as more "natural" and less amenable to change. Outsiders become the focus of jokes, criticism, or even hatred. Examples include all aboriginals and incomers, such as the Nuer of Sudan with the Dinka, the Sioux of North America with Europeans, and the British with those of Asian or Afro-Caribbean origin, (notwithstanding that the British are a curious amalgam of aboriginals and incomers developed over many centuries). This sense of identification with a dominant, more "natural" group can occur within groups, as sub-groups or classes within a group generate these attributions. An example here is the caste system of the Indian sub-continent. A sense of "rightness" or "naturalness" regarding one's own perceptions and feelings can make it very difficult to accept another's, though different, as equally valid.

Identity

Group identity, the result of such attributions, has three components: cognitive, evaluative, and emotional, according to Tajfel (1978). The same author identifies a difficult psychological problem for members of minority groups, that of conflict between a satisfactory self-realization and the restrictions imposed on them by that very membership. Self-image is based on group identity, and comparisons with other groups and individuals play an important part too. Such identity problems can occur as early as six or seven years of age (see Jahoda et al., 1972, re the children of Asian immigrants in Scotland). Identity problems can mean the devaluation of national and ethnic groups, (Tajfel et al., 1972, in Scotland; Lambert et al., 1960, with French-Canadians). However, a pride in membership in the minority may result if there is strong group identity and integrated values, norms, and structures within the minority group.

Values

The values involved in individual and group identity concern the nature of life, man's place in nature, relationships between people, and such processes as birth and death, religion, diet, hygiene, and health. There is often a complex interaction between these values, and the inter-relating system that results can impose tremendous strains when cultural boundaries are crossed (see Mayor, 1984a, 1984b, and Parmar, 1985, for a discussion of such value systems among their Asian clients in England). This is at its most destructive when it involves individuals and their sense of personal identity. Feeling as one with a group, and feeling of value and worth with such identification, individuals have much to lose if this is rejected. A failure to appreciate or to reflect a client's sense of value or worth, as in an empathic response, can have a negative rather than a neutral effect.

SELF-IMAGE

Self-image and self-esteem are closely related and both involve aspects of in-group, out-group bias and group identity. The quality of interpersonal relationships is largely determined by the respective conditions of the participants' self-image and self-esteem. During childhood the developing individual's self-concept is being influenced mainly by parents, other close relatives (siblings, grandparents), and teachers. These significant others, by the examples they set, and by the reinforcement that they give, are powerful agents of growth and development. At adolescence, however, different significant others play an increasingly important role in the burgeoning self-concept. These include peer group members, and others, from a variety of reference groups. In the multicultural setting this can lead to conflicts which are quite complex.

Different models offered by different reference groups, particularly if crossing cultural boundaries, can make it difficult for the development of an individual client, which reduces the possibility of empathy being accurately rendered or perceived.

In many cases the helper is involved because of problems the client experiences with self. Empathic responses are required if such difficulties are to be tackled and growth of self is to be achieved. Even though the helping interaction may take place in a muticultural setting, the problems of self-image or esteem may not be related to cross-cultural factors but to "normal" difficulties associated with, say, adolescence, when child–parent conflict can be extreme in many cultures and lead to identity problems in the growing youth. In such conflicts, however, cultural ammunition may be used by both parents and the youth (see Rack, 1983).

For example, rebellious teenagers, more Westernized than their parents, may reject their Asian culture much in the same way that Western teenagers of the 1980s may reject the 1950s values and attitudes of their Western parents. The rejection is of parenting rather than of the values or culture.

The self-image is expressed, however, in a variety of ways, some of which are non-verbal, and some of which the individual may be unaware. Tajfel (1978) has been quoted above as arguing that there are three aspects to group identity. These three aspects also can be seen as applying to the self image: cognitive, evaluative, and emotional. It is the expression of this latter which is most likely to be subconscious, at least partly, although the evaluative aspect may be expressed also in non-verbal, unconscious ways. Communication between cultures is affected not only by the obvious factors, language, but also by cultural norms regarding the interpretation of non-verbal aspects. Another factor related to communication is what Brislin (1981) calls "conversational currency" (p. 65), by which he means knowing what topics are proper in conversation or interviews. In some cultures, or even within subgroups of some cultures, it is thought improper for certain topics to be discussed or explored in particular settings. Gender also may be important here in that certain topics may not be thought proper between the sexes. Similarly, age may be a barrier to certain topics. Insensitivity to such senses of inappropriateness may inhibit the development of an empathic relationship. This is particularly so if the helper insists on pursuing or reflecting emotions or reactions at a level of advanced empathy.

COMMUNICATION

Language is the most obvious factor in cross-cultural communication. Although languages may differ, there is evidence that people in different cultures use their languages in the same way and to make the same sort of sense of the world. Cole and Scribner (1973) have reviewed the psychological research in this area, and have acknowledged the importance of the Whorfian hypothesis, that language shapes the thought rather than vice-versa. Even with the use of a translator, it is only people from cultures with linguistic similarities, it is argued, who can effectively communicate their experiences because different languages describe things in different ways. Languages which, for example, have the same root, have a similarity that will facilitate this kind of communication, such as the Romance languages, or some groups of American Indian languages. Cole and Scribner, however, point to the inconclusive nature of the research and allow only that there may be some influence of relativity. They refer to Bernstein's work (1972) on the effects of culture on grammatical codes and semantic expression, although the latter has been subjected to some criticism.

An empathic response from a helper assumes a similarity in reactions and meanings, whatever the style of expression. However, the evidence does seem to be that people from different cultures do react emotionally in the same way and give the same kind of meanings to their experiences, however different those experiences may be, and however differently they may express them. However, if someone is living among people of a different culture and language, then the inability to express emotions and meanings can lead to a sense of isolation, whatever the universality of the emotions and meanings. This can lead to a self-centered and idiosyncratic view of reality which the helper may have difficulty in relating to and reflecting (Rack, 1983).

Some cultures, and even subcultures, do not have the words to express certain feelings or meanings. Examples are the rich vocabulary in European languages regarding subjective experiences, whereas in the language of the Yoruba in Ghana there are very few, but in contrast there is a rich vocabulary regarding cattle and familial relationships. This is where education and literacy also play a part. Rack quotes the research of Berger and Mohr (1967), which demonstrated that a subculture, the English working class, did not have the words to translate their knowledge and feelings into thoughts, and thus a great deal of their experience remained unnamed for them, and as a result was difficult to articulate to another, except in non-verbal ways. Rack (1983) also argues that such inarticulation leads to a heightened sensitivity to and even dependence on non-verbal communication. The verbally articulate helper must not be unaware of such modes of experience and communication, acknowledging the often vital importance of the non-verbal in communicating empathy.

Emotional expression may also be subjected to cultural norms and even rituals. Littlewood and Lipsedge (1982) see two levels of expression, private and public. Within a culture, they argue, it is possible to distinguish between them, but across cultures this may be difficult. Effective helpers, sensitive to such levels of expression, will know with which level they are empathizing, and be able to communicate this insight as well.

The use of interpreters or linkworkers can perhaps be helpful in overcoming language deficiencies. Rack (1983) is an ardent advocate of the employment of such facilitators, arguing that they should be specially-trained personnel, rather than children or other relatives or friends, so that they can understand the import of questions. There have been some interesting pilot schemes established recently in the U.K. (Bahl, 1984; Davidson, 1985; Mays & Levick, 1985; Watson, 1986). These projects have been concerned mainly with the Asian community, although one exercise involved Asian and Afro-Caribbean clients (Webb, 1981). In Canada, Jones and van Amelsvoort Jones (1986) have studied communication patterns in the care of the elderly, including immigrant Canadian-born and Anglo-born clients, and have found significant differences in the observed interaction. They recommend the use of translators and the employment of staff who have similar ethnic roots as the client group. The exploration of the client's experiences demands insights into cultural and subcultural dynamics. The problems of the appropriateness of topics, gender, age, ritualistic norms, as discussed above, are much more readily sidestepped or are "inside" the culture and "inside" the helping profession. Responses supported in this way are much more likely to be perceived as empathic by the client.

Some research has been undertaken which suggests that there may be cultural differences in the expression of emotional experiences, particularly in the psychiatric context (see Davis, 1986, for a discussion of the issue of culture and psychiatric nursing). Brown, (1974) has described such differences as found with American Indian groups. She argues, however, that such differences are superficial, that is, lexical rather than reflecting differences of experience. Depression seems to be a particularly problematic emotion. An international survey (Murphy, Wittkower, & Chance, 1964) showed a wide variety of expressions/symptoms, with only four being universal: insomnia; a mood of dejection; social withdrawal; and fatigue. Guilt, a common symptom/expression in Western cultures, was not prevalent in many others. There seemed to be religious connotations involved, with Christian-Judeo cultures being more likely to express intrapunitiveness. This stresses the importance of a thorough exploration of the experiences and reactions as seen by the client in order that responses and reflections are perceived as accurate.

Where verbal language fails it becomes much more important to take note of the non-verbal communications that always occur. Brislin (1981) refers to the vast literature dealing with transcultural non-verbal impression formation and communication. He notes the analysis of such behaviors as the use of space, gestures, clothing, eye contact, facial displays, body positioning, body odors, and conversational style in transcultural interactions (see reviews by Harper, Weins, & Matarazzo, 1978; and LaFrance & Mayo, 1978). Custom and ritual often demand more of non-verbal behavior than they do of verbal, and the potential for cultural influence and transcultural confusion is therefore the greater. This can affect the way in which the client perceives the helper and the way in which the helper perceives the client. This obviously has direct relevance to the perceived accuracy of responses at the verbal or non-verbal levels which are intended to be empathic.

CLIENT PERCEPTIONS OF THE HELPER

The way in which clients see the helper can be related to their self-image, and the points made above are relevant here also. It is the client's perception that determines whether or not a helper is empathic or not.

Role changes imposed on an individual entering or encountering a new culture can influence the self-image and subsequently the way in which other people are seen. Culture shock occurs when the psychological cues that help an individual to function in society are withdrawn or replaced by new ones. The dangers and difficulties of this phenomenon have been researched with reference to the education and training of nurses, in a monocultural context (e.g., Kramer, 1974). One hopes that this insight can be readily transferred to the transcultural context. In many cultures the role of helper often has hierarchical or authoritarian implications and leads to the expectation that such a helper will give instructions and prescribe, rather than the approach that is needed in a counseling or therapist role. In a counseling role the emphasis is on facilitation of client insight and client self-generated growth and development, and for this empathy is essential.

As a defense against the culture shock clients may be experiencing, they may show a variety of behaviors in reaction to the approach offered by the helper, including anger or suspicion. These behaviors may be expressed at the non-verbal level, and may even degenerate into withdrawal from the relationship, psychologically or physically (Osborne, 1976).

Within any culture there is a system of balances which relates stresses, with supportive behaviors and rituals as counterbalances. Examples are mourning rituals to help people cope with bereavement, and rituals associated with birth, adolescence, and marriage. This is related to the discussions on the appropriateness of topics, and the difference between public and private expressions of emotion. Recognition of such stresses as expressed in a particular culture, and the expectations of behaviors and rituals that may accompany them is an important part of an empathic response. Failure to offer or appreciate valid coping strategies will lead to failure of acceptance as a helper (Webb, 1981).

HELPER PERCEPTIONS OF THE CLIENT

The area of the helper's perception of the client has been reviewed, in the nursing context, by Kelly and May (1982) from a sociological standpoint, and by Davis (1984) from a psychological standpoint. Both consider a wide range of research reports which demonstrate the perceptions that the nurses have to certain patients and the difficulties that they have in maintaining an individualized approach to care. The research reviewed included the following kinds of influence: favoritism associated with the nature of the client's problem; romantic and idealized expectations of clients and of the caring role; client's reactions to their problems, whether demanding and complaining, or understanding and grateful; a willingness to accept a dependent role in relation to the nurse. Nurses seem to have stereotyped perceptions of patients and seem to deal with patients as members of a category or class rather than as individuals, as mentioned above.

Osborne (1976) has identified two major errors in nurse–patient relationships in the transcultural context. These are (a) an attempt to be liberal and to ignore the client's cultural identity, dealing as a result with a generic human being, and (b) being overwhelmed by the racial characteristics and dealing with a cultural stereotype rather than the individual. Similar errors have been reported also in Britain (Wilson, 1978; Webb, 1981). Given the points considered in the section on the social psychology of interpersonal relationships above, and as reviewed in more detail in Davis (1984), it can be argued that it would be remarkable if nurses or other helpers did manage to deal with their clients as individuals, showing empathy. There is also much research indicating that in many instances it does not occur (Johnson, 1976). However, many patients or clients do feel that they have been treated or cared for in an understanding way, as an individual, and with a great deal of insight. In spite of themselves and of the system some helping professionals do achieve the remarkable. The questions is, can this approach be made more predictable, more certain?

It has been discussed in earlier chapters that empathy skills can be measured and can be learned. It has also been demonstrated elsewhere that an increase in cultural sensitivity can be achieved in the preparation of nurses, and presumably other helpers (Davis, 1986). Many schools of nursing in North America now incorporate workshops or learning modules into their curricula to increase sensitivities to cultural differences, as described by Branch (1976), Leininger (1978), Baker and Mayer (1982), and Wong and Wong (1982), for example. The latter two examples are particularly useful models because of their experiential nature involving structured interactions.

CONCLUSIONS

Empathy skills are a part of the general armory of helping professionals, along with any other clinical skills which they must employ. Moving into the transcultural setting is adding an extra dimension to those skills, and to the nature of the assessment of client need that the helper makes. An extra dimension is also being added to the self-image of professionals and to their identity as caregivers and as persons. By extending the role of helper into the transcultural setting, practitioners are extending and developing themselves. Personal growth is being experienced. Without the ability to grow and develop oneself, to explore alternatives, one cannot really begin to facilitate such changes and explorations in clients.

The purpose of this chapter is to indicate some of the practicalities of empathy in the helping relationship. This book is concerned with boundaries between theory and practice. Within the various arenas of practice there are also boundaries to be crossed. Cultural boundaries are an important aspect of the structure of most societies today, and no helping practitioner can function in a cultural vacuum. It is hoped that this chapter has shown that cultural sensitivity can be life enhancing for the client, the helper, and for the society within which they live.

REFERENCES

Bahl, V. (1984). Forging a new partnership (interview with Yasmin Alibhai). *Nursing Times, 80*(37), 19–20.
Baker, C. M., & Mayer, G. G. (1982). One approach to teaching cultural similarities and differences. *Journal of Nursing Education, 21*(4), 17–22.
Berger, J., & Mohr, J. (1967). *A fortunate man: The story of a country doctor.* Harmondsworth: Penguin.
Bernstein, B. (1972). Social class, language, and socialization. In S. Moscovici (Ed.), *The psychosociology of language.* Chicago: Markham.

Branch, M. (1976). Models for introducing cultural diversity in nursing curricula. *Journal of Nursing Education, 15*(2), 7–13.

Brink, P. J. (1976). *Transcultural nursing: A book of readings.* London: Prentice Hall.

Brislin, R. W. (1981). *Cross-cultural encounters.* New York: Pergamon.

Brown, M. S. (1974). Anthropology, nursing, and mental health. *Journal of Psychiatric Nursing and Mental Health Services,* 12(1), 7–11.

Burrows, A. (1983). Patient centered nursing care in a multiracial society. *Journal of Advanced Nursing, 8,* 477–485.

Chapman, A. J., & Jones, D. M. (1984). *Models of man.* Leicester: British Psychological Society.

Cole, M., & Scribner, S. (1974). *Culture and thought.* Toronto: John Wiley.

Davidson, N. (1985). Championing minority groups. *Health and Social Services Journal, 95,* 550–551.

Davis, B. D. (1981). Social skills in nursing. In M. Argyle (Ed.), *Social skills and health.* London: Methuen.

Davis, B. D. (1984). What is the nurse's perception of the patient? In S. Skevington (Ed.), *Understanding nurses.* Chichester: John Wiley.

Davis, B. D. (1986). Culture and psychiatric nursing. In J. Cox (Ed.), *Transcultural psychiatry.* London: Croom Helm.

Dobson, S. (1983). Bringing culture into care. *Nursing Times, 79*(6), 53–57.

Egan, G. (1986). *The skilled helper.* Monterey: Brooks/Cole.

Harper, R., Weins, A., & Matarazzo, J. (1978). *Non-verbal communication: The state of the art.* New York: John Wiley.

Johoda, G., Thomson, S. S., & Bhatt, S. (1972). Ethnic identity and preferences among Asian immigrant children in Glasgow: A replicated study. *European Journal of Social Psychology, 2,* 19–32.

Johnson, M. (1976). Communication of patients' feelings in hospital. In A. E. Bennett (Ed.), *Communication between doctors and patients.* Oxford: Nuffield Provincial Hospitals Trust, Oxford University Press.

Jones, D. C., & van Amelsvoort Jones, G. M. M. (1986). Communication patterns between nursing staff and the ethnic elderly in a long-term care facility. *Journal of Advanced Nursing, 11,* 265–272.

Jones, E., & Davis, K. (1965). From acts to dispositions: The attribution process in person perception. In L. Berkowitz (Ed.), *Advances in experimental social psychology (Vol. 2).* New York: Academic Press.

Kelly, G. A. (1955). *The theory of personal constructs.* New York: Norton.

Kelly, M. P., & May, D. (1982). Good and bad patients: A review of the literature and a theoretical critique. *Journal of Advanced Nursing, 7,* 147–156.

King, I. M. (1971). *Towards a theory for nursing.* New York: John Wiley.

Kramer M. (1974). *Reality shock: Why nurses leave nursing.* St. Louis: C. V. Mosby.

LaFrance, M., & Mayo, C. (1978). Cultural aspects on non-verbal communication: A review essay. *International Journal of Intercultural Relations, 2*(1), 71–89.

Lambert, W. E., Hodgson, R. C., Gardner, R. C., & Fillenbaum, S. (1960). Evaluation reactions to spoken languages. *Journal of Abnormal and Social Psychology*, *60*, 44–52.

Leininger, M. (Ed.) (1978). *Transcultural nursing: Theories, concepts, practices.* New York: John Wiley.

Littlewood, R., & Lipsedge, M. (1982). *Aliens and alienists.* Harmondsworth: Penguin.

Mayor, V. (1984a). The Asian community: No. 1, The family, bereavement and dietary beliefs. *Nursing Times, 80*(23), 40–42.

Mayor, V. (1984b). The Asian community: No. 2, Pregnancy, childbirth and child care. *Nursing Times, 80*(24), 57–58.

Mays, N., & Levick, P. (1985). When maternal instinct isn't enough. *Health and Social Services Journal, 95*, 870–871.

Miller, G. A., Galanter, E., & Pribram, K. H. (1960). *Plans and the structure of behavior.* New York: Holt, Rinehart & Winston.

Murphy, H. B. M., Wittkower, E.D., & Chance, N. W. (1964). A cross-cultural enquiry into the symptomatology of depression. *Transcultural Psychiatry Research Review, 1*(15), 5–18.

Osborne, O. H. (1976). Unique needs of ethnic minority clients in a multi-racial society: A psychological perspective. In *Affirmative action towards quality nursing care in a multiracial society* (Publication M-24 2500). Kansas City: American Nurses Association.

Parmar, M. D. (1985). Family care and ethnic minorities. *Nursing—the add-on Journal of Clinical Nursing, 2*(36), 1068–1071.

Peplau, H. E. (1952). *Interpersonal relations in nursing.* New York: G.P. Putnam's Sons.

Pocock, D. (1975). *Understanding social anthropology.* London: Hodder & Stoughton.

Rack, P. (1982). *Race, culture and mental disorder.* London: Tavistock.

Roy, C. (1970). Adaptation: A conceptual framework for nursing. *Nursing Outlook,18*(3), 42.

Tajfel, H. (1978). *The social psychology of minorities.* London: Minority Rights Group.

Tajfel, H., Jahoda, G., Nemeth, C., Rim, Y., & Johnson, N. B. (1972). The devaluation by children of their own national and ethnic groups: Two case studies. *British Journal of Social and Clinical Psychology, 11*, 235–243.

Watson, P. (1986). Towers of Babel? *Nursing Times, 82*(3), 40–41.

Webb, P. (1981). Report of an ethnic health project, 1979/1980. *The Health Education Journal, 40*(3), 69–74.

Wilson, A. (1978). *Finding a voice.* London: Virago.

Wong, S., & Wong, J. (1982). Problems in teaching ethnic minority students. *Journal of Advanced Nursing, 7*, 255–259.

12

Overcoming Barriers to the Use of Facilitative Empathy In Practice

Jean R. Hughes
E. Joyce Carver

The importance of empathy in the helping relationship has been demonstrated in earlier chapters of this text. The means for developing and/or enhancing this dimension in the learning laboratory have been examined as well (see Chapter 8). However, despite the success of empathy training, the transfer of this skill from the safety of the classroom to the realities of the clinical area is fraught with difficulties (see Chapter 9).

Barriers to the application of empathy in professional practice can be grouped into two categories: learning needs and performance problems. Chapters 6 and 8 examine some of these constraints in relation to personal characteristics and the logistics of skill acquisition. This chapter concentrates on the performance problems associated with the professional issues of role perception and situational norms. Implications for the education of future health professionals are suggested, together with recommendations for consideration.

Review of the literature, discussions with the study nurses and an examination of the field notes maintained throughout the empathy research program (Part 3), indicated a number of barriers that potentially inhibit empathy transfer. These barriers were grouped in two interrelated categories: (a) role perception including the professional's sense of image, risk-taking, and control; and (b) situational norms including the elements of environmental expectations, support, and reinforcement. The dimensions within each group will be presented in a manner to illustrate their connectedness.

ROLE PERCEPTION

How a role is perceived is crucial to the credibility of a discipline. With the number of professions in the health care system having mushroomed in recent years, a sense of confusion and competition concerning the delineation of roles with their associated responsibilities has been created. In particular, nurses are unclear about role expectations in terms of their relationships with patients (La Monica, 1983). Some "lack confidence in their profession and in themselves and consequently have a lowered self-esteem" (George & Larsen, 1988, p. 68). Not surprisingly, beliefs about the nurse–client relationship range from the purely social contact to the purposeful and progressive encounter.

Those disciplines whose professional image does not permit engagement may be reluctant to use the skill of empathy as it forces involvement in a relationship beyond the superficial level. In fact, Toi and Batson (1982) found that those who demonstrate low empathy seem to direct their helping behavior to decrease their *own* distress. Those having high empathy show a high rate of helping behavior directed toward the altruistic goal of reducing *client* distress.

Haggerty (1985, pp. 297–298) observed that some professionals hesitate to explore client concerns out of fear of probing, and consider empathy to be unethical. It is recognized that an element of risk-taking is required to translate into practice a role perception that focuses on progressive interaction with clients. Szalita (1976) suggested that some professionals may be hesitant to use empathy if their compassion encompasses much pain and resentment. Distancing serves as a protection for their vulnerable feelings causing anger and a desire to have the client, "out of the way" (p. 151). Further, La Monica, Madea, and Oberst (1987) cautioned that motivation and readiness are important factors to assess in a professional's use of empathy. It may be an erroneous assumption that all "learners want to be facilitative communicators" (p. 210).

Aspy (1975) identified that some professionals believe learned empathy actually detracts from the spontaneity of a helping relationship. They think that helping is a mystical process rather than a deliberate application of learned skills. These professionals often resist the skill of empathy because they do not know how to use it and will not seek assistance "despite their authentic desire to help clients" (p. 13).

Friedrich, Lively, and Schacht (1985) noted two kinds of performance problems with empathy: (a) fear of risk-taking, and (b) premature challenging. That is, they believe professionals either hesitate to encourage the client to focus on problem exploration or show impatience with relationship building and expect to see change occur too quickly. Haggerty (1985, pp. 297–298) identified a number of similar obstacles in the learning process with students. Some respond automatically instead of empathically because of high anxiety, while others have difficulty articulating their thoughts. Both approaches directly affect their interventions.

The issues of fear and control appear to be closely related and present significant barriers to role perception and performance. Professionals may feel helpless to assist clients and therefore, choose to "reassure, teach, advise, and perform physical care when further exploration is indicated" (Haggerty, 1985, p. 298). Clearly the perceived loss of power could be a critical deterrent to the use of empathy. Osterweis, Solomon, and Green, (1984, p. 20) suggest that professionals who set unrealistically high expectations for themselves withdraw and avoid exploring issues with clients. They may be feeling total responsibility for the well-being of those in their care and react out of fear of being identified as failures. Mauksch (cited in Menikheim & Meyers, 1986) has termed this behavior blame-avoidance. The fear of making a mistake is so strong that professionals can never be responsible for a wrong act; "there is an extreme desire to be safe and correct" (p. 83).

Clearly the professional's perceptions regarding the matter of responsibility and its relationship to empathy warrants further investigation in a helping relationship. Our experience supported much of what is reported in the literature. Empathy challenged the nurses in our study to question, and removed their sense of stability. At times it took great willpower to commit themselves to the learning process and absenteeism occurred if the nurses were not up to the emotional investment required. When overcome by the agony experienced by patients, these learners expressed feelings of guilt for their own non-facilitative interaction.

The nurses were reluctant to use empathy if they believed it to be too direct and specific. They needed to appear genuine to the patient, but in the early stages of empathy development they felt phony and mechanical which increased their resistance to the skill. Such fear of risk-taking was demonstrated by repeating questions or reviewing issues previously addressed. Their deliberate use of non-specific, safe vocabulary conveyed a vague message, thereby preventing confrontation with the patient.

The nurses showed their impatience by moving through a battery of unrelated questions or by giving advice on how to resolve a matter before the concern was thoroughly examined. Some referred clients to other disciplines as a last resort, when approaches considered acceptable had failed. These nurses were touched by the distress of their clients, and it would appear the lack of expression of empathy became a measure of professional survival. Interestingly, the nurses stated their awareness of their actions in the training sessions but felt unable to overcome the barriers to the use of empathy.

Not all nurses in our program were prepared to assume responsibility for helping. Some resisted empathy and avoided identifying patient concerns, in order to appear in control. They reasoned that as long as the patient problem remained hidden it would be one less worry.

In summary, compromises in image, ethics, confidence, and control can present powerful barriers to the professional in terms of role perception and ultimately the transfer of empathy from the learning laboratory to the practice setting.

SITUATIONAL NORMS

The literature provides many useful observations regarding the impact of the surrounding environment on the professional's use of empathy. Forsyth (1980) questions whether the organizational structure allows the professional, specifically the nurse, to share actively "of oneself in every interaction" (p. 41). She raises several questions about the relationship between professional satisfaction and retention of nurses in the profession. Does professional burn-out occur more rapidly with nurses who have low empathic experiences and ability? Further, Forsyth asks, does the empathic ability of newly graduated nurses increase or decrease with clinical practice? (p. 41) It would appear that the health care system values the completion of tangible tasks. Graffam (1970) wondered what factors might militate against an empathic, helpful response from the nurse (p. 335). She noted that the nurse is given little assistance in persevering in showing compassion (p. 335).

In her response to La Monica's and others' (1987) study on empathy and nursing care outcomes, Rawnsley (1987) suggested that certain practice environments might facilitate the development and expression of professional empathy (p. 216). Indeed, La Monica and her colleagues showed that nurses working with patients having a diagnosis of cancer demonstrated mean scores close to the maximum on the nurse- and client-rated Empathy Construct Rating Scale. Further, these ceiling scores were achieved prior to taking an empathy training program. On the other hand, Brunt (1985) found that within an institution the "setting plays a questionable role in the practice of clinical empathy" (p. 76). That is, high technology areas (such as intensive care units) do not appear to have any more effect on a nurse's use of empathy than low technology areas (such as hospice units). The high tech settings are now considered to have stress factors that differ in nature rather than intensity from low tech settings. Regardless of the environment, Mynatt (1985) cautioned that "the realities of and stress in the work setting may decrease the level of empathy as a protective device for the nurse" (p. 345).

Kramer (1977) described the work environment of recently graduated nurses as a proving ground. She identified the importance of empathy development in supervisors to enable the achievement of expectations of both the bureaucratic environment and the new professional. She suggested that an accepting climate helped to ensure that the professional felt wanted and prepared for the realities of the work world. The environment must be empathic in nature and project the same qualities to professionals as they in turn are expected to offer in a therapeutic helping relationship with clients. A non-evaluative, accepting atmosphere enables professionals to have a caring attitude toward themselves. Being listened to makes it possible for professionals to listen more accurately to themselves with greater awareness of their visceral experience. According to Rogers (1975) a greater understanding of the self opens up new facets of experience which become a part of a more accurately based self and enhanced ability to be empathic.

Haggerty (1985) noted that many students do not identify positive client outcomes resulting from their interactions and therefore lack immediate feedback and ultimately lack an indication of the effectiveness of nurse–client communication. Guttman and Haase (1972) discussed the importance of reinforcement for ensuring retention of professional empathy skills in the clinical area and clarified that empathy was less subject to extinction, if contingent upon consequent patient behaviors rather than supervisor reinforcement. Friedrich, Lively and Schacht (1985) found that student behavior-specific feedback was important for instructors to give in the early stages of empathy development. However, encouraging students to observe for themselves the positive effects on patient behavior reinforced continued use of empathy in the clinical area.

A number of sources noted the impact of modeling on the support and reinforcement for empathy (for example Layton, 1979; La Monica, 1983; Payne, Weiss & Kapp, 1972; Perry, 1975; Steibe, Boulet & Lee, 1979). Mynatt (1985) observed that students choose role models who have similar empathy levels, weakly suggesting that students tend to be like their teachers. La Monica (1976) believes those who are in authority (e.g., administrators) have a responsibility to practice empathy, as subordinates cannot be expected to maintain a caring attitude for clients in a workplace that mitigates against it. It is recognized that other characteristics, such as clinical competence, expert knowledge, technical skills, and ability to teach effectively may influence professionals' choices of role models too (Mynatt, 1985), however the point is made that models in the environment do seem to have some influence on a professional's behavior.

The nurses in our program identified many similar concerns as those indicated in the literature. They noted the environmental stress factors endured on a daily basis. They felt torn between the demands of the bureaucratic structure of the institution and the patient needs for individualized professional care. The nurses experienced further competition between the instrumental (physical care) and affective (psychosocial) requirements of the patient. On a busy unit the reality of nursing practice often translated into meeting basic survival needs. The constant enforcement of pain on patients, through the debridement of burns or during dressing changes, created a unique form of stress to endure in their work environment. Therefore, any attempt to add an empathic dimension that encouraged patients to elaborate and explore their concerns was overwhelming and at times seemed sadistic. This caused tremendous guilt, frustration, distress, confusion, and anger; all common feelings which contribute to the high turnover rate in the profession of nursing (Duldt, 1981; Baumgart, 1988).

Group support provided a catalyst to the progress of participants. As the nurses identified professional vulnerabilities and anxieties they exposed their interaction skills to each other. For the first time many learned to request feedback and seek assistance from colleagues. Peer consultation has received little attention in nursing until recently. The skill of cultivating relationships to exchange information and resources, commonly known as networking (O'Connor, 1982), together with the mentoring phenomenon whereby a senior nurse helps a younger colleague negotiate the barriers in the workplace (Donner & Hardy, 1988), have begun to make an impact on this process (George & Larsen, 1988). It is hoped that these support systems will aid in the transfer of empathy to clinical practice.

An associated element of informal individual support was found to be important in empathy transfer. The possibility of being ridiculed by colleagues prevented some nurses in our program from testing new dimensions of empathy in the workplace. As they often practiced in close proximity to their peers, they were hesitant to interact with patients using approaches with uncertain outcomes. Private encouragement from a respected colleague proved to be an important reinforcer and was often given by fellow program nurses when other planned physical interventions were being discussed. As well, a positive patient response, most often confirming the nurse's remarks, encouraged the nurse to continue her empathic approach thus establishing reinforcement from the client's perspective.

Our program nurses were more likely to practice empathy if trusted authority figures encouraged its use, or better yet, modeled it themselves. Forsyth (1980) states that "patients ascribe expertise and power to professionals whom they perceive in control" (p. 41). This phenomenon was also noted in the laboratory between the nurses in the empathy training program and the teacher, who was challenged to prove her credibility by demonstrating consistent empathic behavior. Once convinced, the nurses committed themselves more fully to the learning process.

In summary, the importance of situational norms cannot be underestimated in terms of the impact on empathy transfer in practice. Environmental expectations, as well as support and reinforcement available to professionals, clearly influence their decision to use empathy.

IMPLICATIONS FOR EDUCATION

The issues noted above warrant careful examination to determine implications for education of future helping professionals. Gladstein and Rochester (1977) suggested that until the matter of definitions is clarified, specific suggestions for practicing professionals and educators cannot be made. Stone (1982) supported a comprehensive approach to the teaching of interpersonal skills, one that is responsive to "consumer needs, social benefits and conceptual and professional development" (p. 450). Considering the complexity of this task, solutions are unlikely to be forthcoming in the near future. In the meantime the preparation of professionals must continue.

What are some of the elements that could confront the barriers to empathy practice and serve as a foundation for a training program? In terms of role perception, Natale (1972) demonstrated that critical thinking training was an effective method for increasing accurate empathy of first-year university students. It was suggested that those who are encouraged to explore and solve problems are in a better position to learn about the experience of another. Such an approach might promote self-confidence and lessen the anxiety of professionals who are hesitant to use empathy because of competing role demands or fear of peer reprisal.

Szalita (1976) examined those areas that might enhance the learning of empathy. She suggested that students need to cultivate personal awareness and critical thinking skills to react to the sensitivity of the sufferer rather than the magnitude of the misfortune. These skills might be encouraged through the examination of life experiences and the capacity to combine imagination with stored memories and new activities. One of the barriers to the transfer of empathy is the overwhelming impact of the disclosures of some patients on professionals. It may be that the integration of self-awareness activities in empathy development programs could assist students to recognize how the exploration of personal concerns enhances personal insight and therefore their resilience. Such an effort might in turn decrease the threat of exploration with others.

In terms of role responsibility Bath and Calhoun (1977) argued that facilitative level empathy skills be mandatory for entry in the helping professions. Such a requirement would indicate a commitment to a fundamental dimension of the helping relationship and educational programs would have a specific mandate regarding expectations for terminal behaviors.

The importance of performance criteria addresses the transfer barrier of professional role perception. Perhaps if standards for empathy skill were clearly defined students would not wrestle with ambiguous role demands in the clinical setting. Avoidance of the exploration of patient concerns or an automatic referral of these to other professionals would not be tolerated. Similarly, administrators would have to provide adequate staffing to ensure that both the psychosocial and physical needs of the patient were met. The fear of ridicule by peers that frequently prevents professionals from using empathy might decrease if its integration were a clear expectation in the workplace.

In terms of aptitude, the literature makes some interesting observations on the matter of student selection. Carkhuff (1969b) believes that a positive relationship exists between pretraining skill levels and progress made during training. Steibe, Boulet and Lee (1979) demonstrated that successful trainees of state empathy were more easily differentiated and predicted, in particular on the basis of youth. That is, the young learner might be more receptive to skill acquisition than an older learner and have fewer established non-facilitative behavior patterns. As well they showed that "trait empathy was somewhat influential in predicting state empathy" (p. 44).

Hogan (1975) on the other hand commented that the distinction between trait and state empathy may not be relevant because they both have "the same consequences for the client. What counts is whether the counselor acts as if he or she understands a client's expectations and cares about the client's welfare" (p. 17). Presumably this behavior would be impossible to determine without some criteria for measurement. These findings suggest that further investigation is necessary regarding student selection on the basis of age and trait empathy.

In terms of the barriers regarding the situational norms related to environmental expectations—support and reinforcement— clearly training programs must provide an opportunity to practice outside the safety of a simulated clinical environment to enable empathy skill transfer. In his discussion of teacher preparation, Aspy (1975) cautioned that it was not enough to make this group empathic and that indeed it might be negligent if a practical experience in the actual work setting were not included. Presumably the same caution would hold true for other helping professions.

Guttman and Haase (1972) developed a micro-interaction model for teaching empathy. They suggested that before any behavioral training can occur it is crucial to have identified (a) client behaviors which are consistent with a positive outcome of the encounter, and (b) counselor behaviors which lead to those client behaviors. This sequence would ensure that reinforcement be expressed by the client rather than being contingent on an external source such as a supervisor. The approach might focus the role of supervision more appropriately on the provision of global problem-solving consultation, rather than concentrating on immediate feedback regarding isolated interventions on a micro-level.

Hills and Knowles (1983) found that nurses who engaged in supervised practice scored significantly higher in terms of empathy and respect than nurses without supervision. Not defined was the term supervision and not examined was the continuation of these skills with its removal. Apparently, supervision could serve as an important reinforcement for empathy transfer if the users had clear expectations for its role.

Payne and colleagues (1972) examined the kinds of assistance required by different levels of learners in the development of empathy. They observed that the consultative role of supervision became useful to students only as they advanced through the learning process. They suggested that the beginner needs didactic and experiential learning opportunities, while the more advanced student requires consultation in addition to practice activities. Early learning necessitates that the teacher devote more time in the clinical setting to telling the student what to do. Perhaps this type of help would lessen the fear students report of not knowing how to explore issues with patients. They would have the security that the teacher was immediately available, that learning could take place in stages, and hence feel a sense of control over their professional practice. As students progressed, the teaching–learning process could advance through discussion on a consultation basis following practical experience in the clinical area. In this way the development of empathy would be carried out with acknowledgement of the barriers to the transfer process, and students would have the appropriate kind of assistance readily available as their learning needs changed.

In conclusion, it would appear that trainer-related factors such as reinforcement, feedback, support, consultation, and paced learning as well as learner-related factors such as critical thinking and self-awareness have some impact on the transfer of empathy in the clinical area. In our opinion greater emphasis should be placed on a number of areas in future programs for empathy development. These ideas are summarized as recommendations for the reader's consideration:

1. Students in the helping professions should have the opportunity to explore role expectations and associated implications for the projection of a professional image.
2. Learners should be encouraged to develop risk-taking behaviors that permit a sense of confidence, and overcome the need to control and to be perceived as perfect.
3. Educational programs should address the different types of supervision neccessary for beginning and advanced learning.
4. Specific strategies, including a commitment from the clinical areas, should be created for the systematic transfer of empathy to the practice setting.
5. The clinical environment should provide resources to enable professionals to meet psychosocial needs of the client in addition to those of a physical nature.
6. The workplace should foster the development of consultative relationships among professionals, and should position role models in settings to allow modeling behaviors to be nurtured.

SUMMARY

The transfer of empathy from the security of the laboratory to the realities of professional practice presents both learning needs and performance problems. Professional issues related to role perception including image, risk-taking, and control present interpersonal dilemmas, while situational norms including expectations, support, and reinforcement present interpersonal barriers to the practice of empathy. These factors have implications for the education of future helping professionals.

Although the approaches to ensure the permanent transfer of empathy are as yet unconfirmed, a number of strategies have been suggested and have been given some preliminary attention. It is incumbent on professionals in the field to continue this exploration to shed further light on possible solutions.

REFERENCES

Aspy, D. N. (1975a). Empathy: Let's get the hell on with it. *The Counseling Psychologist, 5*(2), 10–14.

Aspy, D. N. (1975b). Helping teachers discover empathy. *The Humanist Educator, 14*(2), 56–63.

Bath, K. E., & Calhoun, R. O. (1977). The effects of professional counselor training on empathy: Continued cause for concern. *Counselor Education and Supervision, 17*(2), 98–106.

Baumgart, A. J. (1988). The nursing work force in Canada. In A. J. Baumgart & J. Larsen (Eds.), *Canadian Nursing Faces the Future*, (pp. 39–61) Toronto: C. V. Mosby.

Brunt, J. H. (1985). An exploration of the relationship between nurses' empathy and technology. *Nursing Administration Quarterly, 9*(4), 69–78.

Carkhuff, R. (1969b). *Helping and human relations, Vol. II: Practice and research.* New York: Holt, Rinehart and Winston.

Donner, G. J., & Hardy, L. K. (1988). Career development and mobility in nursing workplaces. In A. J. Baumgart & J. Larsen (Eds.), *Canadian Nursing Faces the Future* (pp. 297–312). Toronto: C. V. Mosby.

Duldt, B. (1981). Anger: An occupational hazard for nurses. *Nursing Outlook, 29*(9), 510–518.

Forsyth, G. L. (1980). Analysis of the concept of empathy: Illustration of one approach. *Advances in Nursing Science, 2*(2), 33–42.

Friedrich, R. M., Lively, S. I., & Schacht, E. (1985). Teaching communication skills in an integrated curriculum. *Journal of Nursing Education, 24*(4), 164–166.

George, T., & Larsen, J. (1988). The culture of nursing. In A. J. Baumgart & J. Larsen (Eds.), *Canadian Nursing Faces the Future*, (63–74). Toronto: The C. V. Mosby Company.

Graffam, S. R. (1970). Nurse response to the patient in distress-development of an instrument. *Nursing Research, 19*(4), 331–336.

Guttman, M. A. J., & Haase, R. F. (1972). Generalization of microcounseling skills from training period to actual counseling setting. *Counselor Education and Supervision, 12*(2), 98–108.

Haggerty, L. A. (1985). A theoretical model for developing students' communication skills. *Journal of Nursing Education, 24* (7), 296–298.

Hills, M. D., & Knowles, D. (1983). Nurses' levels of empathy and respect in simulated interactions with patients. *International Journal of Nursing Studies*, 20(2), 83–87.

Kramer, M., & Schmalenberg, C. (1977). The first job. . . . A proving ground: Basis for empathy development. *Journal of Nursing Administration*, 7(1), 12–20.

Layton, J. M. (1979). The use of modeling to teach empathy to nursing students. *Research in Nursing and Health*, 2, 163–176.

La Monica, E. L. (1983). The nurse as helper: Today and tomorrow. In N. L. Chaska (Ed.), *The nursing profession: A time to speak*, (pp. 489–499). Toronto: McGraw-Hill Book Company.

La Monica, E. L., Carew, D. K., Winder, A. E., Haase, A. M. B., & Blanchard, K. H. (1976). Empathy training as the major thrust of a staff development program. *Nursing Research*, 25(6), 447–451.

La Monica, E. L., Madea, A. R., & Oberst, M. T. (1987). Empathy and nursing care outcomes. *Scholarly Inquiry for Nursing Practice: An International Journal*, 1(3), 197–213.

Menikheim, M. L., & Meyers, M. W. (1986). Communication patterns of women and nurses. In D. K. Kjervik & I. M. Martinson (Eds.), *Women in health & illness: Life experiences and crises* (pp. 80–87). Toronto: W. B. Saunders Company.

Mynatt, S. (1985). Empathy in faculty and students in different types of nursing preparation programs. *Western Journal of Nursing Research*, 7(3), 333–348.

Natale, S. (1972). *An experiment in empathy*. Windsor, Berks: National Foundation for Educational Research in England and Wales.

Osterweis, M., Soloman, F., & Green, M. (1984). Roles of health professionals and institutions. In M. Osterweis, F. Soloman, & M. Green (Eds.), *Bereavement: Reactions, consequences and care* (pp. 220–234). Washington, D.C.: National Academy Press.

O'Connor, A. B. (1982). Ingredients for successful networking. *The Journal of Nursing Administration*, 12(12), 36–40.

Payne, P. A., Weiss, S. D., & Kapp, R. A. (1972). Didactic, experiential, and modeling factors in the learning of empathy. *Journal of Counseling Psyhology*, 19(5), 425–429.

Perry, M. A. (1975). Modeling and instructions in training for counselor empathy. *Journal of Counseling Psychology*, 22(3), 173–179.

Rawnsley, M. M. (1987). Response to "Empathy and nursing care outcomes." *Scholarly Inquiry for Nursing Practice: An International Journal*, 1(3), 215–219.

Rogers, C. R. (1975). Empathic: An unappreciated way of living. *The Counseling Psychologist*, 5(2), 2–10.

Stone, G. L. (1982). Evaluating the effectiveness of skills training programs. In E. K. Marshall, D. Kurtz & Associates (Eds.), *Interpersonal Helping Skills* (pp. 447–467). San Francisco: Jossey-Bass Pub.

Streibe, S. C., Boulet, D. B., & Lee, D. C. (1979). Trainee trait empathy, age, trainer functioning, client age and training time as discriminators of successful empathy training. *Canadian Counsellor, 14*(1), 41–46.

Szalita, A. B. (1976). Some thoughts on empathy. *Psychiatry, 39,* 142–152.

Toi, M., & Batson, C. D. (1982). More evidence that empathy is a source of altruistic motivation. *Journal of Personality and Social Psychology, 43*(2), 281–292.

13

Empathy: Theory And Practice Issues

Ruth C. MacKay
E. Joyce Carver
Jean R. Hughes

The exploration of empathy as discussed in this book has revealed seven issues which stand out as particularly important.

1. Conceptual agreement concerning empathy as a phenomenon is lacking.
2. The diversity of approaches to the measurement of empathy has restricted opportunities for investigators to build upon the work of others.
3. Empathy can be learned as a skill, but it is quite another matter for skills to be transferred from a laboratory setting into the practice area.
4. The empathic personality predisposition of helping professionals needs further documentation. Particular attention should be directed toward its relationship with state empathy in establishing a therapeutic climate for client care.
5. The significance of empathy in human relations has been clearly reported, but the costs of systematically introducing empathy into the organizational structure of client care agencies as a legitimized expectation for the quality care of clients has yet to occur.

6. The impact of the professional's use of empathy on client wellbeing has just begun to be examined empirically.

7. Theory explaining the impact of empathy on the promotion of client wellbeing is tentative, fragmented, and largely untested.

We shall discuss each of these in turn.

CONCEPTUAL ISSUES

There is no doubt that there is a lack of consensus on what empathy is, how it may be defined, and consequently how it can be measured. Three major schools of thought predominate: (a) empathy is a behavior, (b) empathy is a personality predisposition, and (c) empathy is experienced emotion. This wide divergence of thought has created a plethora of definitions for empathy, each directed to viewing empathy in terms of one particular conceptual orientation. Moreover, measurement of empathy has subsequently and logically followed these varied conceptualizations.

One consequence of this intellectual disharmony has been to slow the development of theory which explains empathy and its impact on therapeutic interaction. Theory and research have been entrenched quite clearly within the boundaries of separate conceptual domains and excursions into neighboring camps have been few. Until there is greater unity of thought in conceptualizing empathy with the achievement of valid and reliable means of measurement, there will be delays in developing cohesive theory in this field of inquiry, and theory for use in practice will suffer accordingly.

THE MEASUREMENT OF EMPATHY

There are unanswered questions concerning the validity of a number of the measures published for assessing empathy. For example, client perception of the helping professional's empathy does not correlate highly with empathy as observed. Furthermore, clients tend to rate professionals as empathic, which is at variance with the fact that this correlates highly with client satisfaction and only to a limited degree with empathic training. Additionally, professionals themselves are biased self-raters, viewing themselves as more empathic than what is demonstrated in practice. The personality component of empathy appears to be tangled in the measurement process with the ability to offer empathy, reflecting the conceptual disharmony already discussed.

Interrater reliability of independently judged empathy is difficult to achieve. There is confusion in determining the exact limits of a unit for measurement from recorded interaction. Then the rating of the unit, once identified, requires judgment again, indicated by the need for a fairly substantial training period in using the behavioral referents established.

Accountability in professional practice requires assessment of the communication skills for helping professionals, with empathy as a component of this. Valid and reliable measurements are prerequisites.

LEARNING TO USE EMPATHY

Educators and helping professionals have demonstrated the effects of empathy training programs on the abilities of practitioners to use empathy. The variety of programs described in the literature show differences in: objectives, the nature of the learner, the characteristics of the teacher, instructional modalities, program setting, and in evaluation.

Objectives of training programs differ widely, ranging from an expectation that trainees will increase their sensitivity to clients and their problems, to a full-fledged ability to prepare practitioners who can offer empathy in an intense client-focused therapy situation. There is a difference, educators point out, between training the ear to hear and the tongue to talk. Is the program to be aimed at increasing the sensitivity of all who come in contact with the client in a practice setting? There are programs which focus on lay counsellors who can listen to others in a helpful manner. Others describe sophisticated long-term programs for counseling psychologists. Still others fall in the middle range, directed at assisting helping practitioners to gain skill in using facilitative communication while giving clients needed physical care. There is one factor on which educators agree: Persons who teach empathy skills must be able to use high levels of empathy themselves, as trainer skill is found to be highly correlated with the outcome ability of the trainees (Carkhuff, 1969, Vol. I, pp. 155–157).

Programs vary widely in length and focus, of course, depending on their objectives. Teaching modalities also differ. Although most programs include an experiential or laboratory component which allows the trainee to practice newly-developing skills, two factors appear to be crucial for gaining and maintaining competence. One is an opportunity for trainees to critique their own skills in an educationally supportive context, such as through viewing a video playback of interaction with a client in a small group learning situation. The other factor is sustained monitoring and feedback in the practice setting until such time as empathy skills are incorporated into the professional's usual communication style. This last factor is difficult to provide in many client care settings where the focus of practice is task rather than process oriented. The transfer of empathy skills demonstrated in the laboratory to the practice setting remains a major problem which has yet to be solved.

Increased need to provide tangible evidence of professional interpersonal competence to meet the requirements of quality assurance programs, accreditation standards, promotional processes, and the professional's self-evaluation, calls for a reliable, valid, and practical measure of interpersonal ability. Review of instruments now available suited for use in clinical situations reveals a void. There is urgent need for development of instrumentation for evaluating facilitative communication in practice settings.

EMPATHIC BEHAVIOR

At this time evidence seems to point to the fact that personality predisposition plus skill in the use of empathy equals empathic behavior of a helping professional. Johnson as well as Gazda and Evans have made it clear that the truly empathic helping professional needs first of all the predisposition to act helpfully as well as training in the skills of demonstrating empathy. In Chapter 4, Johnson has inferred that perceptiveness and compassion, as themes, are requisite for the enactment of empathy in human relations. He notes also the need for a sustained training period with the objective of developing congruence between the helper's intrinsic motives in a client situation and empathic behavior. The acknowledgment that these two different components are linked in the enactment of empathy in helping relationships is indeed a milestone in the study of empathy.

As yet the research literature gives little documentation of how personality and training in skills interact in a clinical situation. It is essential for practitioners to use empathy genuinely; the mechanical use of empathy skills in isolation is insufficient. Personality variables, such as perceptiveness and compassion, need to be included in assessments of empathic behavior and their influence considered in creating a therapeutic environment.

There is a further question to ask in establishing the precise relationship between the helper's personality and skills in producing empathic behavior. Is there a critical point in a scale, which could be developed to assess perceptiveness and compassion, below which a person cannot be properly trained to offer genuine empathy? If in the future this indeed can be identified reliably and validly, such a finding would carry great relevance to policy formation in the admission of candidates to educational programs for the preparation of helping professionals.

THE SIGNIFICANCE OF EMPATHY IN PRACTICE

Educators agree that students need to invest both time and effort in gaining skills in offering facilitative empathy. These commodities necessarily are converted into costs, both for the student and for the educational program. There is a further cost. Many agencies employing helping professionals have a majority of staff who are as yet unable to offer empathy at a facilitative level. Their educational programs either did not include training in the development of empathy skills, or skills gained were not transferred later into the practice area. Thus norms for the expected behavior of staff in facilitative communication in the agency environment may not be high. The results of this can be two-fold. Staff joining the agency may be subjected to pressures from the majority to conform to normative styles of professional–client interaction which do not recognize high levels of empathy. Secondly, if it should be offered, there is no reinforcement for using facilitative empathy from role models or other practitioners, which can have a long-term deleterious effect on continued high-level ability. This points to the need for staff development programs to raise the level of facilitative empathy of practicing professionals together with permanent structures for reinforcement to ensure its use. Costs for such programs could be high. The more important question to ask, however, is what are the costs in patient wellbeing if staff do not gain skills in facilitative communication?

EMPATHY AND CLIENT WELLBEING

So far the evidence from reported research showing the impact of empathic behavior on client wellbeing is limited. A number of reasons have been put forward in explanation. Investigators have been caught up in the conceptual dilemma of defining and measuring empathy, and thus research findings have been relative to particular conceptual orientations. This has diminished effort directed toward a global approach and slowed the accumulation of research findings. Secondly, for many helping professionals there is limited contact with any one client over time. In the hospital setting patient stays are often short, and shift work and team approaches to patient care create discontinuous contacts. Under these conditions it is difficult to identify patient care outcomes which could be directly attributable to the professional's use of empathy. This is probable in some other types of client care environments as well.

The need for focused research attention on the examination of effects of the professional's use of empathy on client care outcomes is critical. Until it is reliably demonstrated that empathy affects the quality of client care there is little justification for educators to include empathy skill attainment in programs for the preparation of helping professionals, nor for managers to support the establishment of staff development and reinforcement programs for this purpose in agency settings. Research evidence needs to include both quantitative and qualitative documentation of results, and to include multicultural implications of the findings as well.

THEORY DEVELOPMENT

A model of empathy was put forward in Chapter 6 as a tentative step toward explaining empathy in professional–client interaction. Research examining conceptual linkages between various sets of variables has been discussed in Chapters 3, 4, and 5 of this book. Research undertaken in the Burn and Plastics Unit and described in Part Three addressed some parts of this model, shown here in Figure 13.1. The model, however, is largely untested.

There is no doubt that in the past conceptual fragmentation in the study of empathy has hindered the development of practice-related theory. However, statements in Chapters 4, 5, and 6 of this book by Johnson, Gazda and Evans, and MacKay, Hughes, and

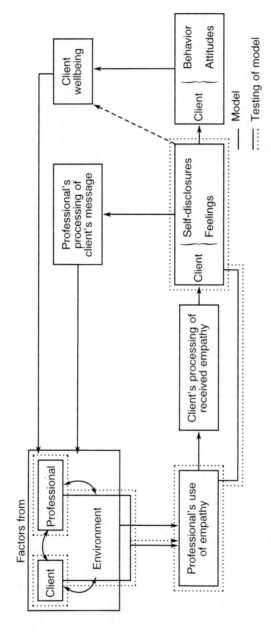

FIGURE 13.1 Testing of parts of the model of empathy in professional client interaction.

Carver, suggest that a broader view of the factors determining empathy in professional–client interaction holds promise of more clearly revealing the intricacies of interrelated factors which describe the helping relationship. Increased recognition of the conceptual complexity of empathy is a first step. The use of multifaceted constructs of empathy in theory development and testing is a further step. There is hope ahead of a more unified approach to theory development in the field of empathy research.

REFERENCES

Carkhuff, R. R. (1969). *Helping and human relationships: A primer for lay and professional helpers*. Vols. I & II. New York: Holt, Rinehart & Winston.

Index